"Why I Became an Occupational Physician" and Other Occupational Health Stories

T0177648

"Why I Became an Occupational Physician" and Other Occupational Health Stories

Edited by

John Hobson
Honorary Lecturer in Population Health
School of Health Sciences
Manchester University
Editor of *Occupational Medicine* 2002–2018

and

The Society of Occupational Medicine

Supporting occupational health
and wellbeing professionals

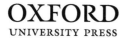

OXFORD
UNIVERSITY PRESS

Great Clarendon Street, Oxford, OX2 6DP,
United Kingdom

Oxford University Press is a department of the University of Oxford.
It furthers the University's objective of excellence in research, scholarship,
and education by publishing worldwide. Oxford is a registered trade mark of
Oxford University Press in the UK and in certain other countries

© Oxford University Press 2020

The moral rights of the authors have been asserted

First Edition published in 2020

Impression: 1

Published in the United States of America by Oxford University Press
198 Madison Avenue, New York, NY 10016, United States of America

British Library Cataloguing in Publication Data

Data available

Library of Congress Control Number: 2020933098

ISBN 978–0–19–886254–3

Printed and bound by
CPI Group (UK) Ltd, Croydon, CR0 4YY

Foreword

"Why I Became an Occupational Physician" and Other Occupational Health Stories is a love letter to occupational medicine, or rather a series of love letters with many authors written over 50 years.

Like many occupational physicians I came into the specialty in mid-career and mostly by accident. I felt a little insecure about that. However reading the series "Why I became an Occupational Physician", I realised rather than being an outlier, my story was not untypical. I was actually part of the 'norm'. This book reflects the diversity of occupational medicine, with professionals from many different backgrounds and experiences all united by a love for their specialty. This eclectic mix of knowledge and experience allows us as occupational physicians to address the myriad of different issues that confront us on a daily basis. If we don't know the answer, we probably know somebody who will.

In this book I learnt of doctors who went on to achieve in different areas of human endeavour, such as Che Guvevara, and Sócrates the Brazilian footballer. There are also stories about some of the greats of medicine: Manson, Thackrah, Legge, and Hunter. Their achievements and their paths were not always easy but they persevered. Their work has had major impacts on the health of workers globally and continues to do so.

I can remember many of these articles when they were first published. I looked forward to the misadventures of Dr Kieran, and hoped I would avoid his pitfalls. I enjoyed reading the history of industry and medicine not only in the UK but globally. Some of the issues faced by our colleagues 50 years ago demonstrates how much things have changed, and depressingly how some of the same problems still challenge us.

I find this book inspiring, informative, and entertaining in equal measure. If I was reviewing for the journal I would rate as a "buy, read, and keep". Put it on the bedside table to give you some inspiration in the small hours.

Dr Will Ponsonby
President, Society of Occupational Medicine

Preface

I fell in love with medical journals and medical journalism as a medical student. Richard Smith was at the *BMJ* and I met him as a third year whilst at a medical student journalism event. I was in awe of what he did at the *BMJ* and some of his ideas truly transformed medical practice throughout the world. I read the *BMJ* voraciously but by far my favourite thing was the filler articles; they even called them that. Here was an incredible insight into the human face of medicine, a relief from the p values and confidence intervals and the scientific straightjacket of evidence-based medicine. Here were amazing tales and wonderful observations, brilliant writing, hilarious or sad, mind-bending and thought-provoking. The fillers were hidden away in the bowels of the journal or in unexpected places, but they made the journey from the front cover to the back an even more interesting one—pleasant punctuations in a panoply of research prose.

When I became Editor of *Occupational Medicine*, it didn't take long for me to realise that perhaps we could have fillers as well. Nerys Williams was even more determined than I was to obliterate the white spaces at the end of research papers and so our series of filler articles began. At first it was mainly a series of articles about why a doctor became an occupational physician, but soon we began to attract pieces from some brilliant writers: Mike Gibson, John Challenor, Nerys Williams, and of course the superlative Anthony Seaton, amongst others. Their pieces are all here along with a selection of some of the other filler articles the journal has published. But perhaps the greatest achievement of the *Occupational Medicine* filler was to record the reasons why almost fifty doctors became occupational physicians, a unique record of why people enter a unique speciality. They are all collected in this book. You can read about whether this was a 'Road to Damascus' moment, or something that just happened, or an event that triggered a realisation that here was an area of medicine that provided something very different. My favourite remains the account by Bill Gunnyeon, which has the honour of starting the book but I am sure you will have your own favourite or discover another.

Enjoy the book. It has been a long time in the making but I am sure you will agree that it has been worthwhile, and if anyone ever wanted to understand what makes an occupational physician tick, they need look no further.

John Hobson

Acknowledgements

The Editor and Society of Occupational Medicine would like to pay special thanks and acknowledgment to the authors of the original articles, namely:

Ken Addley
Folashade Adenekan
Raymond Agius
John Aldridge
Eric Altschuler
Roy Archibald
Simon E. Asogwa
Ralph Aston
Alan Bailey
B.S. Baker
Eva Baranyiová
Dianne Baxendine
Jerry Beach
A. O. Bech
J.J.A. Blakely
Naomi Brecker
Monty Brill
Tim Carter
Clodagh Cashman
John Challenor
Arun Chind
D. Coggon
Richard Colman
Morris Cooke
Karen Coomer
Joan M. Davies
Stephen Deacon
Joshua Devonport
William M. Dixon
Arthur Eakins
Hans Engel
Ian Reid-Entwistle
Jean Spencer Felton
Ann Fingret
Timothy Finnegan
David Fishwick
Giuliano Franco
John Garnett

Malcolm Gatley
Kirstie Gibson
Mike Gibson
W. Glass
Henry N. Goodall
Roy Goulding
Paul Grime
Bill Gunnyeon
Timo Hannu
Graham Hardy
Peter Harries
Vanessa Hebditch
Athol Hepburn
Emma Hirons
John Hobson
D.L. Holness
R.W. Howell
G.O. Hughes
J.A. Hunter
William R. Jenkinson
Tomoyuki Kawada
Joseph L. Kearns
M. D. Kipling
Frank Klont
G.L. Leathart
Kenneth Lee
Gary Liss
Stewart Lloyd
A.C. Mackay
Ira Madan
D. Malcolm
R. Ian McCallum
Paul McKeagney
Mike McKiernan
J.T. Mets
John D. Meyer
Elizabeth Mitchell
Syed Nasir

Desmond O'Neill
L.G. Norman
B.H. Pentney
James Preston
John Rich
A.W.W. Robinson
Susan A. Robson
Anthony Ryle
Hanaa Sayed
Douglas Scarisbrick
Anthony Seaton
Chris Sharp
Gordon Shepherd
Andy Slovak
David Snashall
John Sorrell
John Storrs

Ian S. Symington
P.J. Taylor
Eric Teasdale
F. H. Tyrer
Katherine M. Venables
Peter Verow
C.A. Veys
R. Viner
David Walker
Robert Willcox
Nerys Williams
Paul Williams
Sabine Wicker
Barbara Wren
David Wright
H. Beric Wright
W. E. Zundel

Contents

Why I became an occupational physician …

Bill Gunnyeon

I often wonder if perhaps it really all began on 22 February 1953 on a hillside in Fife close to RAF Leuchars from where a short time earlier my father, at the controls of a Meteor jet, had taken off never to return. Less than 4 months later I entered the world. I do not recall as a child ever expressing a desire to be a pilot or being especially interested in flying; and as the time came closer to making a career decision, I felt somewhere deep down that I wanted to study medicine. Transferring schools for my final year, my new rector peered down his nose at me during our first meeting and with a sneer pointed out that I would be lucky to get into university let alone medical school. So it was with unashamed haste that my unconditional offer from Dundee University was accepted.

Freshers Week introduced us to all the opportunities for engaging in anything but study and here I came across the University Air Squadron—and suddenly I knew I had to join and learn to fly. East Lowlands Universities Air Squadron was clearly very gullible and before I knew it I was being taught to fly a Chipmunk—from RAF Leuchars no less. It quickly became clear that I did not possess my father's natural flying ability but I do have the consolation of having flown solo!

My new found interest in flying led to an interest in all things to do with the RAF which allowed me to convince a Selection Board that I was a good bet as a future RAF Medical Officer; any pecuniary interest in improving the quality of my life at University was purely coincidental! Thus for the second time, the RAF had a Gunnyeon on its list of officers and I experienced the mix of primary care and occupational health from which the first spark of interest in occupational medicine was ignited.

Responsibility for the health of those engaged in a diverse range of occupations during three tours of duty on operational flying stations (and yes I did get to fly in a Lightning); a year's involvement with the rehabilitation of bandsmen of the 1st Battalion Royal Green Jackets after the bombing in Regents Park in 1982 and a chance encounter involving some alcohol and a discussion about the Worshipful Society of Apothecaries Diploma in Industrial Health fanned the flames of my interest in the specialty—and the rest as they say is history!

Was my ultimate destiny just a series of unconnected coincidences? Was there something about flying inherent in my make up destined to bring me into contact with the RAF and expose me to occupational health? Or was there some greater hand influencing and shaping my future? Who knows? I often wonder though if my father would have approved of my career choice—I hope he would.

Source: *Occupational Medicine*, Volume 57, Issue 2, March 2007, Page 84, https://doi.org/10.1093/occmed/kql099. © The Author 2007.

Those extra moments

Jean Spencer Felton

In the move to managed health care, the interaction between the occupational health physician and employee/patient has mimicked somewhat the brevity of the medical visit experienced external to the worksite. Whereas, in former days, there was no sharply predetermined time to be devoted to the individual seeking care, today's hurried schedules usually allow 15 min or less per visit.

Such sharp temporal demarcation allows the ailing person to declare his or her health concerns, a hasty examination by the care provider, the issue of appropriate prescriptions for medication and some counsel concerning the clinical findings, with, possibly, allusion to the patient's inappropriate health-affecting life style. In industry, there may be additional precautions offered concerning the performance of certain job functions in light of the presenting disorder.

While such a visit will meet the physical needs of the patient, rarely are basic emotional, behavioural, family or interpersonal difficulties explored. Yet, it is the underlying problem that is most bothersome to the client and which has had no inquiry. The employee leaves, still burdened by the unresolved dilemma that he or she may not even connect to the presenting ailment.

An invaluable opportunity to be of true assistance to the patient is passed, often not just because of time or schedule constraints, but because of discomfiture felt by the practitioner in the exploration and guidance required by these problems whose etiology may be completely outside the workplace.

It has been the practice of the writer, on completion of the worker's visit, to utilize some extra moments to inquire 'How are things at home?' or 'How are things going on the job?' There is a brief period of silence, followed by a low-pitched 'Oh, that son of mine', or 'Things are not so hot at home.' The door is open, thereafter, to exploration of the true problem troubling the individual and to professional guidance for the rectification of the current dysfunction at home or at the workplace.

An employee was shown his X-ray films as part of a survey of personnel exposed to asbestos, past or present. The findings were explained and reassurance was given as to the minimal changes encountered. On completion of the clinical aspects of the visit, the query was placed regarding conditions at home and the response of 'Oh, my daughter ...' was given. Further questioning revealed that the late teenager had not spoken to her family for many months. It was arranged that she visit the occupational health service for an interview.

It was anticipated that the young woman would be an angry, mute, non-communicative person, with whom interaction would be difficult. To the contrary, on entry, the daughter was bubbling with smiles and energy, talked freely, and welcomed any expressed concerns by her parents. She played guitar, composed music, was highly articulate and willing to have the family situation rectified. Counselling was initiated and communication reinstalled within the family.

On another occasion, on completion of the clinical aspects of the visit, the same question was put to the employee concerning events other than those at the work setting. An extremely concerned response was given regarding a 15-year-old daughter who had a presumably uncontrollable, spasmodic, persistent, non-productive cough (48 coughs per min) and who communicated solely by written notes. She had been studied by 14 specialists at a variety of hospitals without change in the condition. Following the obtainment of records, appropriate referral was made to a university medical center and with indicated clinical tests and psychotherapy, all difficulties cleared. Subsequently, the young woman became a physician.

In all comparable instances the employed parent(s) were extremely grateful for the directive care given and for the lifting of the heavy emotional burdens occasioned by difficult situations away from work. These examples are offered to lend credence to the belief that a few moments of concern about the real problems perplexing workers can be totally rewarding to the occupational health service, the distraught employees' families and to the involved persons themselves.

In a recent 'Piece of my mind' in the *Journal of the American Medical Association*, the author wrote, '[We] physicians are still incredibly blind to a critical area of professional skill—our ability to listen to and talk with our patient. [The] number one complaint from the patients was always the same—they said that far too often we medical colleagues don't take the time to really understand how they feel' [1].

In parallel with this observation is the late Arthur Ashe's comment in his autobiography, that while serving on hospital boards he had 'seen studies of patients' complaints that list at the absolute top the doctors' chronic unwillingness to listen to them' [2].

Practitioners of occupational medicine can readily alter this public view by utilizing those extra moments to seek the true problem behind the patient's need for help. Many a clinical visit is made without the employee's ability to, or being given the opportunity to, express the true underlying quandary that is affecting his or her home and family life and job.

May those few extra moments be used to change some seriously damaged lives and restore well-being to troubled employees and their loved ones.

References

1. Jenkins HS. A piece of my mind—the morning after. *J Am Med Assoc* 2002;**287**:161–162.2.
2. Ashe A, with Rampersad A. *Days of Grace—A Memoir*. New York: Knopf, 1993; 211–212.

Source: *Occupational Medicine*, Volume 52, Issue 6, September 2002, Pages 357–358, https://doi.org/10.1093/occmed/52.6.357. Copyright © Society of Occupational Medicine 2002.

3

One hundred years of the health and safety laboratory 1

Anon

Early in the Second World War, there was a need to improve anti-aircraft shells to help defend Britain against German bombing raids. One problem was that no-one knew how the shells actually broke up when they exploded. Work had been done catching the bits in sandbags and wooden targets, but this didn't show how each part of the shell contributed to the fragment pattern. The Ordnance Board turned to "a very skilled scientific team at our Safety in Mines Research Establishment in Buxton" who developed tests showing the origin of each fragment and how fast it travelled (see Figure 3.1). This allowed mathematical models of shell bursts to be developed, and statistical techniques employed to improve the effectiveness of firing patterns. The SMRE team also went on to develop methods by which the fragment size from these aerial explosions could be more closely controlled, allowing more predictable results.

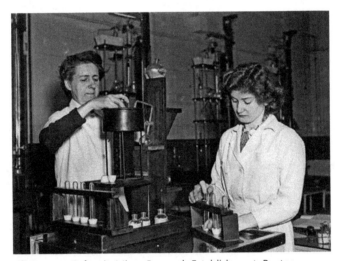

Figure 3.1 Scientific team at Safety in Mines Research Establishment, Buxton
© Crown copyright 2011.

Source: *Occupational Medicine*, Volume 61, Issue 5, August 2011, Page 294, https://doi.org/10.1093/occmed/kqr111. © Crown copyright 2011.

Fifty years ago: 'Raynaud's phenomenon in a pneumatic tool worker'

A.C. Mackay

Syndrome

Raynaud's phenomenon is defined as 'intermittent pallor or cyanosis of the extremities' precipitated by exposure to cold, without clinical evidence of blockage of the large peripheral vessels. First noted in 1911 in users of pneumatic hammers in Rome. Two classes of tools are known to give rise to the condition: (1) those with a to and fro motion of a piston and (2) rotating tools, usually electrically driven.

In December 1935, the mechanical engineer of a locomotive repair workshop received a complaint from a number of men engaged in riveting copper stays. They desired to call attention to the condition of their fingers 'which became numb and useless members of our hands' and which they considered to be due to the use of pneumatic tools. They quoted two examples of the awkwardness caused: (1) difficulty in opening a carriage door and (2) applying the brakes of a cycle. These men had been employed for periods varying from 3–6 years on this work, symptoms having been first noted on an average about 2–3 years after commencing this type of work. The work consisted of the riveting of cold copper stays by means of a light pneumatic hammer. The stays were riveted with the boiler upright so that the riveting hammer was held horizontally against the stay head. The pneumatic hammer itself weighed about 13 pounds, had a bore of just over 1 inch diameter, a stroke of 3½ inches, and delivered blows at a rate of 2,100 per minute.

Dr Hunt examined a number of these men at the neurological clinic at St. Bartholomew's Hospital and later read a paper at a meeting of the Royal Society of Medicine from which I quote:

> The workman grasps the underside of the vibrating end of the instrument with his left hand and the index finger of this hand is always the first to be affected. The cramped position in which the locomotive men work, together with the weight of the tool, forces them to change hands often, and although the fingers of the left hand are those affected first, all the fingers of both hands suffer in the end. It is the hardness and unyielding nature of the cold rivets which is partly responsible for the symptoms of which these men complain, and which other riveters escape.

Attacks of Raynaud's phenomenon appear at first only occasionally, in winter, but later more and more frequently and even in summer. They vary from a slight pallor of one finger-tip to cyanosis and numbness of all the fingers of both hands. The affected fingers are described by the men as 'feeling cold', 'going white', 'waxy', 'numb', or 'dead'. If the cyanosis lasts for more than half an hour the skin of the finger-tips becomes quite anaesthetic and will not bleed if cut. General examination of these men, including investigation of the urine, blood pressure, blood Wassermann reactions revealed nothing abnormal.

History

Mr. H. had been continually employed for over five years on work of this type of pneumatic tool and he first noticed trouble after 13 months which was earlier than the average and this may have some bearing on the severity of his symptoms later. He had to leave this type of work completely and in spite of this had to give up work altogether in May 1952. Various treatments were tried—histamine ionisation, injections of Padutin, but these were only of temporary benefit.

Examination

When I saw him in June 1951 the hands appeared normal but slightly colder than would be expected. As the examination room was exceptionally warm (88°F) the hands were immersed in tap water at a temperature of 68°F. Within a minute blanching commenced at the tips of the fingers and thumbs and although the hands were removed and dried the pallor spread over the whole hand up to the wrists and lasted about 10 minutes before gradually disappearing.

Discussion

The cold immersion test is described as being carried out with the hands immersed in water at a temperature of 59°F for 15 minutes. The rapid release of the circulatory defect in this case at the relatively high temperature of 68°F may perhaps be accounted for by the severity of the condition combined with the high room temperature prevailing at the time.

Source: *Occupational Medicine*, Volume 53, Issue 5, 1 August 2003, Page 342, https://doi.org/10.1093/occmed/kqg078. Copyright © Society of Occupational Medicine 2003.

Originally from: *Trans Assoc Ind Med Officers*, 1953, 3:266–267.

5

Thoughts on lawnmower blades

Anthony Seaton

He was about my age and had left school at 15. 'What was your first job?' I asked. 'Sharpening lawnmower blades; the old-fashioned ones you pushed' he replied. It made me think. It must be 30 years since I did that. When we married 40 years ago, we had a cooker, but no car, washing machine, dryer, refrigerator, central heating, television or vacuum cleaner. My mother brought up her five children without any of these aids and I recall my grandmother, to whose home we were evacuated during the war, cooking in a small oven over an open coal fire. All through my childhood, a coal fire was the source of heating through the winter. We were not poor; this was the norm in the 1940s and 1950s.

The fuel that supplied our energy needs was coal. The coal industry employed about one-tenth of the male UK workforce, and chimneys everywhere belched out black smoke which, during temperature inversions, settled as a dense cloud over the cities and was responsible for many thousands of premature deaths. The major episode in London in 1952 led to the Clean Air Acts. Coal burning was prohibited in cities, power stations moved to the countryside and tall chimneys sent the sulphurous pollution to northern Europe where it acidified lakes and rivers. But the effects on our pollution have been dramatic. Less polluting fuels, more efficient engines, better insulated houses and less energy-dependent industries have allowed us to come close to closing the coal industry and given us the chance to live in a more fuel-efficient manner. All we had to do was to maintain the same austere lifestyle and all would have been well. But we overheat our houses, think nothing of flying away on holiday and drive cars seriously overpowered for our needs. We use fuel to cut our grass, wash everything, watch television, write articles and play games on computers, even to clean our teeth. Every time we do these things, we draw unrenewable energy from the planet and add to the burden of carbon dioxide in the atmosphere.

I believe that the concept of sustainable development is a comfortable myth. Global climate change is a reality and, as atmospheric CO_2 continues to rise, we shall soon reach a point at which climatic changes will affect all those now under the age of 40. Indeed, it may already be too late to do other than mitigate the worst effects. At any time, death of forests and oceanic algae, melting of polar ice and release of methane could accelerate temperature rise, force more crop failures, flooding and drought and lead to further internecine war and migration from hard-hit places. We are entering a period of sustainable retrenchment. The young, who have grown-up accustomed to their parents' profligacy, will find it difficult to adapt. It would help them if we now started to set a better example.

It is funny what lawnmowers make you think of.

Source: *Occupational Medicine*, Volume 58, Issue 6, September 2008, Page 444, https://doi.org/10.1093/occmed/kqn101. © The Author 2008.

6

Why I became an occupational physician …

C.A. Veys

It was towards the end of World War II that the first seeds of my interest in the health of those at work were sown. As a teenager, I used to accompany my father on visits to his factory at week-ends. Barbed-wire, torpedo nets, and the ubiquitous 5-gallon petrol can, found on every jeep and army lorry, were being manufactured 7 days a week. Restrictions imposed by blackout impeded good ventilation, so dust, fumes and also noise abounded. The adversities under which men and women worked prompted my question: 'Who looked after their health?'

In 1950, I applied to Sheffield (my home town), Manchester and Liverpool Universities for a place to study medicine. Initially I was turned down—'too young', was their reply, 'go and do your military service first'. Liverpool, however, were persuaded by my great uncle, Rodhain, Dean of Tropical Medicine at Louvain University in Belgium, at least to grant me an interview. I got in, but throughout the 6-year course little if any mention was made of the diseases of occupation. Donald Hunter's influence had not reached this far north, and his landmark text was only first published in 1955, the year before I qualified.

After a 3-year short service commission in Tanganyika with the King's African Rifles based in Dar es Salaam, I undertook a full-time course in public health. This was on the advice of the British Postgraduate Medical Federation, who suggested that the best way into occupational medicine at that time (1960) was to gain a DPH, then a DIH from within industry working as an assistant industrial medical officer. During the DPH course I was fortunate to be able to visit Hamish Cameron's dynamic unit at Pilkington's Glass Works in St Helens, and that of Richard Trevethick at the giant steelworks of Steel Peach and Tozer in Sheffield. Hamish also ran a transitional work-shop, and Richard a small glove factory for employees returning to work after serious injury or prolonged illness, in order to rehabilitate them back into their normal job, or other suitable work. Both these insights further enhanced my interest in health at work, and my wish to study it.

In 1963 I joined Michelin Tyres in Stoke on Trent, being further nurtured and guided by Ronald Lane and Tommy Scott at Manchester; then by Richard Schilling at the London School of Hygiene and by Bobby Case at the Chester Beatty Institute of Cancer Research—who better as mentors for encouraging a career in occupational medicine.

Now in retirement and looking back over 35 years in a previously rather unexplored industry healthwise, I feel rewarded by a branch of medicine that offered me research combined with day-to-day practice in the factory, and close contact with people at work. I have no regrets at having turned down an offer from Prince John to come back and work among his Masai people on com-pletion of my military service.

Source: *Occupational Medicine*, Volume 56, Issue 1, January 2006, Page 5, https://doi.org/10.1093/occmed/kqi162. © The Author 2005.

Thackrah's grave

Graham Hardy

The Leeds surgeon Charles Turner Thackrah was the first to make a systematic study of occupational diseases, and his premature death deprived the Leeds School of Medicine of one of its keenest intellects and most diligent teachers. His biographer Meiklejohn stated that, despite having searched many records, he had been unable to locate Thackrah's grave [1]. I was fortunate to discover the grave at St John's churchyard, Dewsbury Moor, during a Sunday afternoon walk about 3 years ago (see Figures 7.1 and 7.2).

Dewsbury is an industrial town about halfway between Leeds and Huddersfield. On the western edge of the town is Dewsbury Moor, which overlooks the valleys of the River Calder and its tributary, the Spen Beck. St John's, which was consecrated in 1827, is a substantially unaltered commissioners' church built in a simple gothic style. The architect was Thomas Taylor of Leeds. Thackrah's grave is at the northwestern corner of the churchyard, close to the boundary wall. The stone commemorates Thackrah and his second wife Grace, who was the youngest daughter of Abram and Mary Greenwood of Dewsbury Moor House.

By the time of his second marriage, the bitter and public disputes with his medical colleagues in Leeds were over and Thackrah had been a widower for about 2 years. The wedding ceremony at Dewsbury Parish Church on 8 March 1830 was conducted by the Rev. Dr Martin Naylor of Wakefield, who was headmaster of Wakefield Grammar School, a prominent liberal and freemason, editor of the *Wakefield Star* newspaper and absentee vicar of Penistone. The witnesses were John Beswicke Greenwood, the bride's elder brother, and Henry Yates Whytehead, Thackrah's friend and former pupil.

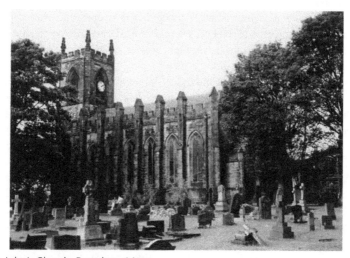

Figure 7.1 St John's Church, Dewsbury Moor.

Reproduced with permission from Hardy G. (2003). Thackrah's grave. *Occup Med (Lond)*. **53**(8):505-6. DOI: 10.1093/occmed/kqg146

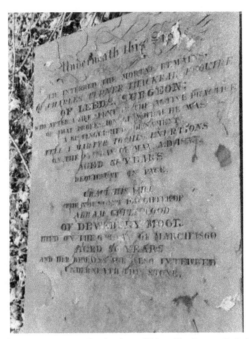

Figure 7.2 Gravestone of Charles Turner Thackrah and his wife Grace. St John's Church, Dewsbury Moor.

Reproduced with permission from Hardy G. (2003). Thackrah's grave. *Occup Med (Lond)*. **53**(8):505-6. DOI: 10.1093/occmed/kqg146

Henry Whytehead was later to write that following his marriage, although Thackrah's bodily health was impaired, the morbid irritability of his feelings was sensibly diminished [2]. Despite his illness, the years that remained were Thackrah's most productive. His great work, 'The effects of the principal arts, trades and professions ... on health and longevity ...', was published in 1831. He wrote a pamphlet on cholera, having visited Tyneside during an epidemic. He accepted an invitation to take part in the foundation of the Leeds School of Medicine and merged his own Anatomy School with the new institution. From its very first session on 25 October 1831, he participated actively in the teaching programme.

Thackrah continued to work for social and industrial reform. He was a principal speaker at the great meeting in Leeds on 9 January 1832 called to express support for Michael Sadler's Factory Bill. The conclusion of his speech 'The proposed measure of limiting the hours of labour is therefore recommended alike by patriotism, justice and humanity' received loud applause [3]. When Sadler introduced his Bill 'for regulating the labour of children and young persons' in Parliament on 16 March 1832, he quoted Thackrah's work at length.

Early in 1833, Thackrah began to prepare a new edition of his textbook on the disorders of the blood. He became ill, however, with pulmonary disease, in addition to the chronic intestinal disorder that had troubled him for almost 20 years, and he died on 23 May 1833, the day after his thirty-eighth birthday. The funeral at Dewsbury Moor took place on 29 May, Dr Naylor coming over from Wakefield to officiate.

Thackrah's epitaph reads 'After a life spent in the active practice of that profession of which he was a distinguished ornament (he) fell a martyr to his exertions'.

References

1. **Meiklejohn A.** *The Life, Work and Times of Charles Turner Thackrah, Surgeon and Apothecary of Leeds (1795–1833).* Edinburgh: E & S Livingstone, 1957.
2. **Whytehead HY.** *Biographical Memoir of C T Thackrah.* 1834. Quoted in Meiklejohn, A Thackrah anthology. Unpublished manuscript, Medical Library, University of Leeds, 1957.
3. *Leeds Mercury.* Leeds City Library, 1832.

Source: *Occupational Medicine*, Volume 53, Issue 8, 1 December 2003, Pages 505–506, https://doi.org/10.1093/occmed/kqg146. Copyright © Society of Occupational Medicine.

Reprinted by permission of Oxford University Press on behalf of the Society of Occupational Medicine.

8

The celebration of Saint Monday

Mike Gibson

A recent mental health case in the clinical examination for the Diploma in Disability Assessment Medicine involved a man whose alcoholism was uncovered by frequent Monday absenteeism. This is widely taught in occupational medicine. An example is in Fitness for Work where it states, 'Markers of misuse include absenteeism, especially on Monday mornings … ' [1]. But for how long has the association been recognized?

The dislike of Mondays amongst the working population is almost universal. Bob Geldof wrote a song in 1979 entitled 'I Don't Like Mondays' and the cartoon character Garfield is known for his dislike of Mondays and liking for strong coffee. Brewer's Dictionary of Phrase and Fable defines Monday morning blues as 'a disinclination to start work after the weekend break' [2]. This source also states that Saint Monday was a facetious name given to Monday because it was observed by shoemakers and other tradesmen as a holiday.

The term 'Saint Monday' is defined in the Oxford English Dictionary [3] as 'the practice among workmen of being idle on Monday as a consequence of drunkenness on the Sunday', commenting that it was chiefly used in the phrase 'to keep Saint Monday'. The earliest quoted source in the Dictionary is in The Scots Magazine for April 1753 in an article entitled 'St Monday; or the tipling (sic) tradesmen'.

However, in 1725, Benjamin Franklin, at that time working as a printer in London, wrote in his diary [4]: 'Those who continued sotting with beer all day, were often, by not paying, out of credit at the alehouse, and used to make interest with me to get beer, *their light*, as they phrased it, *being out*.... My constant attendance, (I never making a St Monday), recommended me to the master; and my uncommon quickness at composing, occasioned my being put upon all work of dispatch which was generally better paid. So I went on now very agreeably'.

So the phenomenon was known at least 280 years ago, although I suspect that it is as old as regular work itself.

References

1. **Smith G, Cook CCH.** Alcohol and drug misuse. In: Cox RAF, Edwards FC, Palmer K, eds. *Fitness for Work*, 3rd edn. Oxford: Oxford Medical Publications, 2000; 480–492.
2. Brewer's Dictionary of Phrase and Fable, Millennium Edition. London: Cassell & Co., 1999.
3. Oxford English Dictionary, Compact Edition. Oxford: Oxford University Press, 1971.
4. **Wright E,** ed. *Benjamin Franklin, His Life as He wrote It*. London: Folio Society, 1989.

Source: *Occupational Medicine*, Volume 55, Issue 5, August 2005, Page 342, https://doi.org/10.1093/occmed/kqi068. Copyright © The Author 2005.

Sócrates

John Hobson

He was named after a Greek philosopher by his self-educated father. He strolled around midfield like a disinterested Greek god, six foot four, bearded, resplendent in the yellow of his country. When the ball came to him he would explode into action, the whole of his team moving like a clockwork machine around him, inevitably, irresistibly moving the ball into the net, usually spectacularly, a feat he managed 22 times in 60 appearances for his country, twice part of the best team never to win the World Cup in the 1980s.

I knew all that, and I can still picture him in action. It was only when reading his obituary that I discovered so many other things about an extraordinary life in and beyond football. He led player's revolts for better terms and conditions; his club's supporters protested about his lack of visible celebration when scoring, something he managed 172 times in 297 matches, and he only played one season in Europe for Fiorentina. He played 12 min for Gosforth Town against Tadcaster Albion in a Northern League game in 2004 when he was reported to be a decade too old to play.

He became a social activist and campaigner for democracy, something that grew out of his campaigning for improved conditions for his team mates, at a time when the oppression by the club management reflected the conditions in the country at large under the military dictatorship. Despite warnings from his national football association, the players wore shirts with 'Vote on the 15th' printed on the back, urging the public to take part in the upcoming elections that were one of the first moves towards ending the dictatorship at a time when people were afraid to speak out against the regime. He was as proud of his team's valiant contribution in helping dismantle the dictatorship as he was of his considerable football achievements. His team won the championship with 'Democracia' printed on the back of their black shirts. It was 'perhaps the most perfect moment I ever lived. And I'm sure it was for 95% of my teammates too.'

He was urged by Gadhafi in a midnight meeting in a tent to stand for president. His childhood heroes included Che Guevara and John Lennon. He smoked and drank beer copiously, which contributed to his premature death at the age of 57; his warm up at Gosforth included two bottles of beer and three cigarettes. He wrote a thesis on the need for fundamental changes to football as a result of players' increasing athleticism, which increased the distance they ran per match from 4 to 10 km in under 30 years. He was one of the few medically qualified doctors to play at the highest level, qualifying from the University of Sao Paulo while playing professional football. He practised medicine after retiring. His nickname on the pitch was 'the doctor'. His name, Sócrates Brasileiro Sampaio de Souza Vieira de Oliveira, MD (19 February 1954–4 December 2011).

Source: *Occupational Medicine*, Volume 62, Issue 5, 5 July 2012, Page 370, https://doi.org/10.1093/occmed/kqs085. Copyright © The Author 2012.

Reprinted by permission of Oxford University Press on behalf of the Society of Occupational Medicine.

Why I became an occupational physician …

Stewart Lloyd

There are one or two colleagues who already know how I became an occupational physician, it being the sort of 'swing the lamp' story that emerges late at night in conference hotels. I was, at the time, a medical officer in the Royal Fleet Auxiliary (RFA) Service, the seagoing arm of the Royal Naval Supplies and Transport Service, an organization that supports the navies of NATO. The job could be very professionally isolated but I was fortunate enough to have the support of my ship-mates and, of course, living cheek by jowl with them, I learnt a great deal about their jobs. Fitness for work was an integral part of the assessments I carried out on the patients who presented at the door of the sickbay and, in common with many small organizations, even if only a few of the crew were incapacitated, this could have a serious effect on the ship's ability to carry out its mission and even compromise its safety.

My ship was on the final stage of the journey home from a long deployment when one of the crew had an acute psychotic episode. We were lucky enough to be going alongside in a Royal Naval dockyard that had a nearby medical centre and, of course, the first thing I did when we docked was call for backup. The ambulance duly arrived and one of the personnel inside it was Surgeon Lieutenant-Commander Geoff Helliwell, RN. A few days after delivering the unwell sailor to the nearest psychiatric hospital, Geoff and I were sitting over a glass or two in the wardroom when the conversation turned to career options. The RFA was great fun, I had seen a fairly good chunk of the world and had some extraordinary experiences, but I did not feel that I wanted to spend the rest of my working life at sea. I was unsure what the future held (except that I was certain that I did not want to go back to the NHS) and, as Geoff was already a trainee in occupational medicine, he suggested that I consider it. I knew next to nothing about it but as we sat and talked about what the specialty involved, I found myself thinking, 'This is what I already do'. Geoff proposed me for the Society of Occupational Medicine and, following acceptance, I attended a few meetings of the London Group. I was then hooked.

Applying for formal training posts was difficult when I was spending up to 8 months of the year at sea but I eventually secured one with British Steel at Scunthorpe, and was lucky enough to have my seagoing experience retrospectively recognized as training time by the faculty. My original NHS career, as an ENT surgeon, also came in handy when dealing with one of the commonest physical hazards in heavy industry, noise.

I have had an 'interesting' medical career, with a number of abrupt right-angled turns and a great deal of serendipity, but I would not swap a day of it for anything else.

Source: *Occupational Medicine*, Volume 56, Issue 3, May 2006, Page 154, https://doi.org/10.1093/occmed/kqj035. Copyright © The Author 2006.

Reprinted by permission of Oxford University Press on behalf of the Society of Occupational Medicine.

'Working Lives' by John Darwell

Anon

This Manchester issue of *Occupational Medicine* features a selection of photographs by John Darwell. 'Working Lives' was commissioned in 1986 by Stockport Museums and Gallery Service as part of 'British Industry Year.' John's aim was to look at the clothing industries around the Stockport area, historically famous as a centre of the hatting industry, but also other traditional industries such as leather production and clog making.

'Looking back on these images from a gap of almost 20 years it seems impossible to imagine such working conditions today; in fact one of the locations is now a museum! As society has changed so have people's workplaces, and interestingly, their physicality. It would be fascinating for me as explorer and documentor to be offered the opportunity to revisit these locations to see what has changed over the intervening period, but perhaps what would be of even more interest would be to see what hasn't.'

John Darwell is an independent photographer working with museums and galleries on projects that reflect his interest in social and industrial change and his concern for the environment. He is a lecturer and researcher on the BA Hons Photography course at the Cumbria Institute of the Arts.

His work has been exhibited in London, Amsterdam, the USA, Mexico, South America and the Canary Islands, and has featured in collections including the National Museum of Photography Film and Television, Bradford, the Victoria & Albert Museum, London and the Metropolitan Museum of Art, New York.

His past projects include 'The Big Ditch' on the Manchester Ship Canal, 'Regeneration' on the demise of the steel industry in Sheffield, 'Scratching the Surface' on the quarries of the English Lake District, plus a trilogy of projects based at locations that have become notorious due to their nuclear connections, including Los Alamos, the Trinity Site, Hiroshima, Nagasaki, Three Mile Island, Sellafield and Chernobyl. He has a forthcoming exhibition and book titled 'Dark Days' documenting the impact of foot and mouth disease around his home in north Cumbria and later this year his book 'A Black Dog Came Calling' will be published. This is an allegorical 'journey' through the process of depression and is being produced as part of John's practice led PhD research into the depiction of depression through contemporary photography.

For further information and to view images from all John's projects please visit his website at www.johndarwell.com. The book of 'Working Lives' is available from Stockport Museums Service.

Source: *Occupational Medicine*, Volume 55, Issue 4, June 2005, Page 250, https://doi.org/10.1093/occmed/kqi102. Copyright © The Author 2005.

Reprinted by permission of Oxford University Press on behalf of the Society of Occupational Medicine.

Fifty years ago: 'Harmful noise'

J.J.A. Blakely

I think it is fair to say that this country is becoming increasingly noise conscious. In America, claims for loss of hearing due to acoustic trauma are common, and one wonders how long we can escape them here. If you enter an environment where, because of the noise, normal conversation is difficult or impossible and you must shout to make yourself heard, then you may be in the presence of harmful noise. It is harmful because it causes deafness by damaging the organ of Corti in the internal ear. This deafness may be temporary, but if it is the result of prolonged exposure, it may be permanent and irrecoverable. Such noise is far from uncommon in industry. Very loud noises can cause permanent damage after a single, short exposure; sharp interrupted noises are probably worse than continuous sounds of otherwise similar characteristics.

Figure 12.1 shows an individual undergoing an audiometric examination in a soundproof room, where the background noise level is as far below 50 dB as possible.

Audiograms should be done on all new entrants who will be working in noise above the 85–90 dB level. Repeat examination in a month will show the susceptible individuals who already have a loss in the higher frequencies; these are the men with 'tin ears', as they say in the States, and they should be transferred to other work. Thereafter the examination can be done six-monthly.

It is not easy to lay down medical standards for noise exposure. If the audiometric survey is adequate, it is probably reasonable to expose many types of individual, provided that at the first sign of deterioration they are moved to safety. However, it would be wise to exclude anyone suffering from deafness likely to be progressive, and who might attempt to claim aggravation. Suppurative

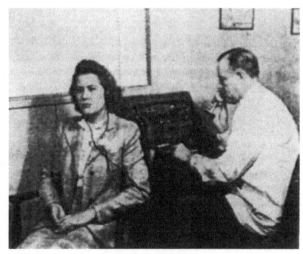

Figure 12.1 Individual undergoing an audiometric examination in a soundproof room, where the background noise level is as far below 50 dB as possible
Reproduced with permission from Blakely J. J. A. (1956). Harmful Noise. *Occup Med (Lond)*. **6**(2):56-59. https://doi.org/10.1093/occmed/6.2.56

otitis media and otitis externa preclude the wearing of ear defenders. Totally deaf people may be exposed, always provided their deafness is not a source of danger.

The duty of the industrial medical officer is clear. He must approach the highest level of management, the level which can authorize heavy costs. To them, he must explain the nature of the noise hazard, and outline his programme to counteract it. After that the decision to proceed lies entirely with management, they must take the responsibility of whether to act now and run the risk of stirring up trouble, or wait until possibly worse trouble is forced upon them. This is perhaps a suitable place to point out that senior executives usually locate their offices in the quietest place!

Source: *Occupational Medicine*, Volume 56, Issue 8, December 2006, Page 589, https://doi.org/10.1093/occmed/kql118. © The Author 2006.

Originally from: *Occup Med (Lond)* 1956; 6.

Tales of Kieran: The occupational physician's odyssey 1—Solvents

J.A. Hunter

I met Kieran at a meeting recently and as it was some time since our paths last crossed we spent half an hour catching up on each other's news. Kieran is the Occupational Physician for Lincaster Health Authority and has an outspoken word on most topics. 'Playing the devil's advocate' he calls it but he invariably ends up in court or on the television which of course as a good Irishman he relishes.

'Solvents' he said after a while. 'Oh yes?' I replied sensing a Kieran-speciality. 'Yes, solvents. I was rung by a solicitor yesterday asking for my expert opinion.' Kieran recognizes himself as an expert in everything from bluegreen algae to electro-magnetic fields so a new expertise came as no surprise. I plugged him further.

'The solicitor represents two octogenarian sisters who have run a small dry-cleaning business for sixty years. They claim the dry-cleaning fluid has caused mental deterioration and they want to sue the company who make the solvent. The solicitor heard I was an expert and sought my services but that is the only sensible thing he has done so far.

'First I asked him whether he had the data sheet on the solvent; he hadn't. Had exposure levels been measured? No. Which neurologist examined the old girls? They hadn't seen one. What were the results of the psychometric assessments, CT scans, EEGs and relevant blood tests? Were they necessary he asked? And no he hadn't approached the manufacturer. He did have a letter from the general practitioner who was sure that their dementia was due to solvent, however.

'When I told him that probably wasn't much use and there was no good evidence that exposure to solvent caused dementia he got quite annoyed and asked if I could recommend any other experts.'

'And did you?'

'Of course. There are three other experts I know but I didn't tell him that two work for the manufacturers and the third is an academic in Japan.'

This all seemed a bit disappointing for Kieran. I'm still waiting for another incident on the scale of the body mass index-at-pre-employment-screening episode. That ended with a confrontation between Kieran and fifty overweight and very angry domestics on live television. He obviously detected my despondency and so kindly reassured me he felt there was bound to be more mileage in this one.

Funnily enough I bumped into Kieran shopping with his wife a few weeks later. 'Any more on the solvents?' I asked eagerly. 'No' came the somewhat muted reply. Then I noticed that Kieran was beardless although it's the first time I have ever seen him facially denuded. His beard has always been his pride and joy especially when stroking it whilst passing some expert comment on television. 'What on earth happened to your beard?' I exclaimed incredulous that I hadn't noticed it sooner. Kieran took a sudden interest in an adjacent tobacconists which is also strange for a man who has an asthma attack when exposed to cigarette smoke. I turned my questions to his wife.

'Kieran managed to stick a carpet tile to his face at the weekend' she obliged. 'The staff at Lincaster General had quite a job detaching him from it.' I was still not much wiser but persisted.

'He was laying carpet tiles in the hall' she explained. 'It went quiet for a long time so I went to investigate and found him unconscious with his face stuck to the floor. The hospital thought he must have been overcome by the solvent in the glue as he hadn't opened the windows.'

I looked around to see Kieran through the shop window about to buy a pipe.

I've decided not to mention solvents for a while at least until Kieran's beard grows back but I am just wondering if that pipe is the first sign of dementia.

Source: *Occupational Medicine*, Volume 52, Issue 2, 1 March 2002, Page 107, https://doi.org/10.1093/occmed/52.2.107. Copyright © Society of Occupational Medicine 2002.

Reprinted with permission from Hunter J. A. (1991). *Lancet*. 337(8753):1341.

Why I became an occupational physician …

Katherine M. Venables

Like others writing in this series, my move into occupational medicine was a change from my original career direction and I have never regretted it. My work has always been varied, interesting and challenging and I relish the opportunities it provides to look at work, workplaces, law, government and all sorts of areas which other medical careers never penetrate.

In the late 1970s, I was making my way up the respiratory medicine career ladder as a medical registrar but had become indefinably dissatisfied. When I failed to get one particular job that I had set my heart on I looked around for alternatives. I brainstormed with anyone who would listen and found a welcome from occupational medicine. I was impressed that senior physicians in the Society of Occupational Medicine and the Faculty of Occupational Medicine were prepared to spend time talking to me. The Medical Women's Federation directed me to Suzette Gauvain whose advice, to get on to an occupational medicine senior registrar rotation, I disregarded. Instead I spent a year as a full-time MSc student at the London School of Hygiene and Tropical Medicine (LSHTM) and thought that I might go back to respiratory medicine.

Once on the LSHTM Occupational Medicine course in 1979–80, I was bowled over by Corbett McDonald's epidemiology teaching and decided that this was what I wanted to do for the rest of my professional life. I found it logical and intellectually satisfying. I also enjoyed being at the inception of disease, with the opportunity of obtaining information which would help to prevent disease. I did my MSc dissertation on the epidemiological detection of occupational asthma with Tony Newman Taylor at the Brompton Hospital, which gave me my first taste of research. After the MSc course, I was offered two complementary jobs, one at LSHTM and one at the Brompton. These gave me tremendous opportunities to carry out research, postgraduate teaching, specialist clinical work and editorial and advisory work. I never moved back to respiratory medicine and have since moved further towards the mainstream of occupational medicine by applying epidemiological principles to research on service provision in occupational health.

In retrospect, I may have been primed by experience of occupational lung diseases as a registrar and by reading Raymond Parkes' wonderful book on occupational lung disorders. My undergraduate experience may also have influenced me: Pat Lawther gave enthralling lectures about occupational diseases and environmental pollution and invited students to his outpatient clinic, from whence they returned with tales of detective work to find out the cause of patients' symptoms. Although we saw it as exotica—rather on a par with the forensic medicine lectures—it is interesting to reflect that we probably had more face to face teaching time on occupational medicine at Barts in the 1960s and 1970s than most UK medical students do today. But the welcome I received from senior members of the specialty as a mere registrar and the high quality of the LSHTM MSc course were undoubtedly the main factors in my decision.

Source: *Occupational Medicine*, Volume 56, Issue 4, June 2006, Page 271, https://doi.org/10.1093/occmed/kqj040. Copyright © The Author 2006.

Reprinted by permission of Oxford University Press on behalf of the Society of Occupational Medicine.

Fifty years ago: 'A Mobile Consulting Room'

G.O. Hughes

The problem of medical examinations for small numbers of employees scattered over a large area has been solved in the North Western Gas Board by the use of a mobile consulting room. The Board has 20 000 employees in an area of 4000 square miles, mainly situated in the counties of Lancashire and Cheshire. There are three fixed examination centres in the area, and works' surgeries at some of the larger works, which are also used for conducting medical examinations. The mobile consulting room is supplementary. This mobile unit has now been in use for just over 12 months. In that time 2974 people have been seen. The medical service is still being built up in the area and the unit is not yet being used to capacity. On a basis of 20 patients per day, and allowing for travelling time, the unit can deal with 5000 patients per annum if it is in use 5 days per week. After a year's working, it can be said that the unit has proved its worth and it is felt that, it could be used with advantage by medical officers who face a similar problem (Figure 15.1).

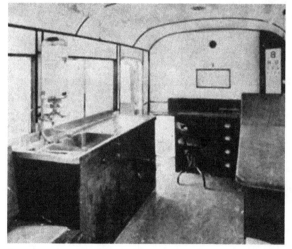

Figure 15.1 Interior view.
Reproduced with permission from Hughes G. O. (2005). A Mobile Consulting Room. *Occup Med (Lond)*. **55**(4):251. https://doi.org/10.1093/occmed/kqi004

Source: *Occupational Medicine*, Volume 55, Issue 4, June 2005, Page 251, https://doi.org/10.1093/occmed/kqi004. © The Author 2005.

Originally from: Report on a Demonstration given at the Annual Provincial Meeting of the Association, Manchester, July, 1954.

Reprinted by permission of Oxford University Press on behalf of the Society of Occupational Medicine.

Excellent credit rating

John Challenor

'Five hand-sets! I've never seen that before'. All the salespersons in the Phones To Confuse U shop crowded around the screen. I had been upgrading my old mobile phone—a friendly brick-sized object that had been a faithful companion for nearly 10 years but could no longer support my new sophistications in communications. I asked what it meant and was there a problem? Far from it, the salesperson said with a totally new deferential manner (did I even detect a sense of awe?) 'It's the highest credit rating we've ever seen in this shop!'

So, here I was in my seventh decade having achieved a five handset credit rating. I did not feel all that different but I did wonder whether this was not a profoundly sad reflection of the state of our credit-riven society. But maybe not. After all, had not I been assigning credit ratings to patients since medical school? The outpatient clinic sister, who had taken a shine to her current batch of junior doctors, would whisper in conspiratorial motherly tones not to take the next patient off the list. 'Look at the size of his notes'—at least four inches thick with a bundle of X-ray films and other assorted investigation that required volumes two and three. Or, 'not that one; they complained about the examination couch being a drab colour last time'.

And so my own system of poor credit ratings has evolved over the years. Patients with more than one volume of clinic notes, patients on a lifelong mission of righteous indignation about all the injustices they have suffered at the hands of doctors, nurses, receptionists, banks, building societies and traffic wardens. But then, there are those with the best credit ratings. Patients and employees who have worked for dozens of years and have wafer thin medical notes. Even when they were crushed by a 50-ton hydraulic platten press and suffered multiple fractures and chronic symptoms of compartment syndrome would limp into my office the day after hospital discharge asking to get back to work. Well good for them. Excellent credit rating.

Source: *Occupational Medicine*, Volume 58, Issue 8, December 2008, Page 579, https://doi.org/10.1093/occmed/kqn103. © The Author 2008.

Reprinted by permission of Oxford University Press on behalf of the Society of Occupational Medicine.

17

Two words and a man

Anthony Seaton

The word 'incentivize' is not in most dictionaries, as it is newly coined to describe the process whereby business people are persuaded to work harder by the incentive of a large bonus at the end of the year. The implication is that they have a job that does not bring its own rewards; that money is the main motivation of their industry. It has recently been used with respect to the learned professions, teachers, doctors and academics. An English Minister of Health has justified his Government's agreement to the consultant contract in terms of the need to incentivize doctors. Why did not this word exist until recently? Because there is another perfectly good word with the same meaning, 'motivate'.

The word 'professionalism' has its roots in the profession of faith and is commonly used to denote two contrasting concepts: the receipt of money by sportspeople and the attitude of a member of one of the learned professions. During the Industrial Revolution, it was characterized as the professional ideal, describing the activities of the doctors and academics, loosely grouped around Jeremy Bentham, whose skills were devoted in a disinterested manner to the service of their fellow man and woman. This understanding of professionalism is what motivated most of us to enter medicine.

Patrick Manson graduated in medicine in Aberdeen in 1865 and, armed with a microscope, went to work in Formosa. He saw many patients with diseases unknown in the West. When consulted by a local mandarin who expectorated onto the floor, Manson scraped the sputum up and examined it under his microscope, discovering the lung fluke, *Paragonimus*. In Amoy, mainland China, he saw many patients with elephantiasis. Isolated and busy, he nevertheless patiently looked for the parasite in patients' blood, finding it came out at night and reasoned that it was transmitted by a nocturnal vector. He fed the blood of a patient to the local *Culex* mosquito and showed that the parasite thrived in its stomach. Thus, he founded medical parasitology and paved the way to prevention and treatment of many tropical diseases. Reasoning that malaria was similarly transmitted, he urged Ronald Ross to dissect the stomachs of mosquitoes to search for the parasite. Ross won the Nobel Prize for this discovery.

Manson went on to found the first western medical school in China and assisted in the foundation of the College of Medicine in Hong Kong. Hoping to retire to Scotland, he returned only to lose his money in a crash of the Chinese stock market. Needing to earn a living again, he set up in practice in London, later founding the London School of Hygiene and Tropical Medicine. Manson's professionalism led to great advances. In his old university, we tried to foster in our students both an interest in the relationships between mankind and our changing environment and a desire to understand and manage the causes of ill-health. We hoped that this would be their motivation and that they would never need incentivization.

Source: *Occupational Medicine*, Volume 59, Issue 1, January 2009, Page 71, https://doi.org/10.1093/occmed/kqn117. Copyright © The Author 2009.
Reprinted by permission of Oxford University Press on behalf of the Society of Occupational Medicine.

Why I became an occupational physician …

John Sorrell

It all started when I was a partner in a rural general practice. It was decided at a partners' meeting one Monday in 1985 that we should all find a clinical assistantship. Our village had a government establishment on its boundary and regularly the Civil Service occupational physician in London requested a medical report about a patient of mine employed there. That Monday I put a postscript on the latest report I had written. 'If you ever need any help locally I might be interested.' Dr Tony Haines, from the Civil Service Occupational Health Service, telephoned me saying he would value some help. Within a few weeks of a pub lunch with Tony I was doing a session a week at this establishment. It took me about three sessions to realize I was out of my depth and knew nothing about occupational medicine. Panic discussions with Tony encouraged me to consider the Manchester Distance Learning Course which I completed and enjoyed enormously, particularly the 'summer school'.

I studied for and passed the AFOM in 1989. The AFOM Journal was a problem, as the government establishment would not give me permission to record my work activities there for security reasons. Cap in hand I approached Eoin Hodgson, who was then medical director of Milton Keynes Occupational Health Service (MKOHS), for help with occupational experience that I could use for my exam journal. Eoin was tremendously supportive and he arranged my contact with a wide range of workplace environments throughout Milton Keynes. I battled on in general practice as a general practitioner (GP) trainer but the sessional occupational medicine was becoming an increasingly important part of my professional life. I had joined ALAMA and SOM and the regular contact with other occupational health colleagues fed my enthusiasm for the subject. I started to do sessions with MKOHS and increasingly felt that I wanted to specialize. Eoin, now at Oxford University, continued to encourage me and in 1994, aged 47 and after 18 years as a GP, I took the plunge and set up as an independent occupational physician. MKOHS was one of my clients and I became their medical director, Eoin agreed to become my supervisor for my specialist training until his untimely death and I eventually became MFOM and accredited in August 2000. MKOHS (one of the original Charitable Occupational Health Trusts) became MKOH (a private company) and the range and diversity of workplaces I became involved with grew rapidly. I still live in the village where I was a GP and not once have I had a twinge of regret about my career change. I feel that the GP experience was a vital background for my current job but the only regret I have is that I did not switch my career 10 years earlier.

Source: *Occupational Medicine*, Volume 56, Issue 5, August 2006, Page 293, https://doi.org/10.1093/occmed/kql006. Copyright © The Author 2006.

Reprinted by permission of Oxford University Press on behalf of the Society of Occupational Medicine.

The Hawthorne effect

Anon

'The consumer of knowledge can never know what a dicky thing knowledge is until he has tried to produce it'; F. J. Roethlisberger, investigator at Hawthorne.

The Hawthorne effect is a familiar anecdote to occupational physicians given that it relates to experiments with improved factory lighting which increased the productivity of workers. Incrementally increasing the level of lighting brought about increased output until someone reduced the level below baseline and output increased still further. The moral of the Hawthorne effect is that people change their behaviour when they think you are watching it and this principle has wider implications in medicine to describe the improved health of control groups.

But how many of us know the origins of the fable? Gale [1] recounts the story and its background in a fascinating piece of occupational medicine archaeology: 'The story relates to the first of many experiments performed at the Hawthorne works of the Western Electric Company in Chicago from November 1924 onwards. The original aim was to test claims that brighter lighting increased productivity, but uncontrolled studies proved uninterpretable. The workers were therefore divided into matched control and test groups and, to the surprise of the investigators, productivity rose equally in both. In the next experiment, lighting was reduced progressively for the test group until, at 1.4 foot-candles, they protested that they could not see what they were doing. Until then the productivity of both groups had once again risen in parallel. The investigators next changed the light bulbs daily in the sight of the workers, telling them that the new bulbs were brighter. The women commented favourably on the change and increased their workrate, even though the new bulbs were identical to those that had been removed. This and other manoeuvres showed beyond doubt that productivity related to what the subjects believed, and not to objective changes in their circumstances. These at least seem to be the main facts behind the popular legend, although these particular experiments were never written up, the original study reports were lost, and the only contemporary account of them derives from a few paragraphs in a trade journal'.

This paper examines the social, political and industrial background to these experiments which took place in a rapidly industrializing United States following the doctrine of Taylor and with huge immigration from Europe to man the factories. The Hawthorne experiments continued for a number of years before the factory collapsed catastrophically in the depression of 1932; Western Electric's turnover reduced from $411 million in 1929 to $70 million and 80% of the workforce lost their jobs. The story looks at the women who were studied (and who became celebrities as a result), the investigators, the academic industry that was born and the wider implications for medicine today. Ultimately, it is the researched who stand out rather than the researchers; five young women entered the folklore of sociology because they got faster and faster at making

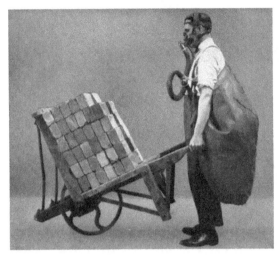

Figure 19.1 Measuring industrial fatigue, 1920s style.
Reproduced with permission from Hill A. V. (1927). *Living Machinery*. London, UK: G. Bell & Sons.

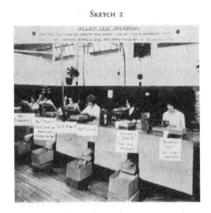

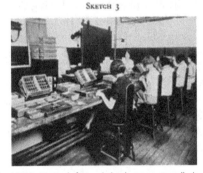

Figure 19.2 The Test Room in 1931. From left to right (upper panel), layout operator, Anna Haug, Wanda Blasejak, Theresa Layman, Jennie Sirchio, Mary Volango.
Reproduced with permission from Gale E. A. M. (2004). The Hawthorne studies—a fable for our times? *Q J Med.* **97**:439–449. https://doi.org/10.1093/qjmed/hch070.

telephone relays (Figures 19.1 and 19.2). Their work also entered the folklore of medicine, as an 'effect' that everyone refers to, but no one can source or define.

The complete article is accessible through the QJM website (www.qjmed.oxfordjournals.org).

Reference

1. **Gale EAM.** The Hawthorne studies—a fable for our times? *Q J Med* 2004;**97**:439–449.

Source: *Occupational Medicine,* Volume 56, Issue 3, May 2006, Page 217, https://doi.org/10.1093/occmed/kqj046. © The Author 2006.

Fifty years ago: 'Free enterprise and public service'

Anon

But what happens with occupational health? The fate of the Slough Occupational Hygiene Service is the latest instalment of a sorry tale of Governmental indifference and the misguided application of a political slogan in this field. It began as part of the Slough Industrial Health Service, and was described in the first volume of this journal (Nash, 1951, 1, 123). Its laboratories were established at the London School of Hygiene, where they remained until 1956, when they were moved to Slough. In 1961, with the assistance of a grant from the Nuffield Foundation, it was established as an independent unit, aiming to serve industry in the whole of the British Isles, and equipped with the men and facilities for investigating and advising on the industrial environment. It had to become self-supporting, by means of the fees charged to industry for its services. In March 1964, it died. It had committed the unforgivable sin of the Admass world—*it was not a commercial success*.

Repeatedly, we have been told that the Government favours the maximum possible voluntary effort in the field of occupational health. What this has meant in effect, both for the Occupational Hygiene Service and for the majority of the group occupational health services which exist, is that having been launched by charity, which is none the less so for bearing a respected name, they must sell themselves to industrialists just as motor cars and television sets are sold to the public. Thus, doctors and their co-workers are forced into a field for which they are untrained and must undertake, in addition to their proper work, a kind of sales promotion which must be amateurish, is distasteful and distracting, and which may at times bring them perilously near to offending against the accepted ethical code, which precludes advertising.

This state of affairs stems directly from Government policy. There are quite genuine practical difficulties in the way of establishing a national occupational health service, even given the will; its financing and its staffing would both present major problems. But no such considerations need have prevented the Government from saving the Slough Occupational Hygiene Service from extinction, either by underwriting its deficit or by taking it over and assigning it to the Factory Inspectorate, which possesses no comparable facilities of its own. Countries with a mere fraction of our population and wealth, such as Finland, put us to shame in this respect, but Her Majesty's advisers were unmoved.

A time is bound to come when we cease to apply the standards of the world of commerce to occupational health services. Meanwhile, tragically, the team is already disbanded, and the equipment sold; but at least the pioneering achievements of the Service will be remembered, and something at least of its experience will reach its successors. Its epitaph should mark its demise as a sacrifice to an economic doctrine applied in a context where it is supremely irrelevant.

Source: *Occupational Medicine*, Volume 64, Issue 2, March 2014, Page 86, https://doi.org/10.1093/occmed/kqt159. Copyright © The Author 2014.

Originally from: Free enterprise and public service (editorial). *Occup Med (Lond)*. 1964;14:1. DOI: 0.1093/occmed/14.1.1.

Adapted by permission of Oxford University Press on behalf of the Society of Occupational Medicine.

Born to Run?

John Hobson

I've never really enjoyed running and yet it is something I have done for most of my adult life. Running is unpleasant, mainly painful, you want it to stop and it's often dark, cold, raining or all three. Motivating yourself to go running can be hard. Who in their right mind would want to get home after a busy day, change into shorts and then a few minutes later feel as if they were about to expire? Perhaps it was cross country running at school having been deemed unsuitable for the rugby pitch. I remember traipsing, lobster limbed, over open moorland in freezing temperatures, howling winds and lashing rain every Wednesday afternoon. The experience must have left deep rooted masochistic tendencies that periodically throughout my life have caused me to pull on running shoes and complete some hellish event such as a 10k, half marathon and for some inexplicable reason, the London marathon. The one time running is enjoyable is when it stops; my only runner's high is akin to not bashing your head against a wall. I do appreciate the benefits of running, the instant stress relief—it's hard to worry about anything when fighting for breath—and the very noticeable improvements in almost all aspects of health and well-being but I've always preferred hill walking as a means of exercise. Unfortunately a hill is a less accessible piece of exercise equipment than a road or a canal towpath. But walking of any type is more enjoyable than running and I don't have many patients who escape advice on exercise, particularly the benefits of walking. So it is interesting to learn that we are designed to run and it should feel very natural to us. In a fascinating *BMJ* podcast [1] Daniel Lieberman, an evolutionary biologist from Harvard, explains how we have evolved to run. Our ancestors started walking 6 million years ago losing the ability to gallop in the process. The ability to run long distances evolved about 2 million years ago and enabled 'persistence hunting'—we run at speeds that make animals gallop which prevents them panting, they have to stop to cool down and we catch them up. The human body is beautifully designed to run. We have short toes, an arched foot and a strong Achilles tendon which together act as a powerful spring mechanism, returning almost 50% of the energy from foot strike. Other features include long legs, a waist that enables us to turn our bodies, semicircular canals that maintain balance while turning our head and crucially millions of sweat glands enabling us to lose heat while running. This evolution is so efficient that, incredibly, running uses barely more calories than walking. A male hunter gatherer covered 15 km a day costing 1000 calories if walking, but only 1400 calories if running. I'll try and remember that the next time I pull those running shoes on or perhaps I'll remember that you don't have to run to burn the calories.

Reference

1. http://www.bmj.com/podcast/2011/11/25/evolved-run

Source: *Occupational Medicine*, Volume 62, Issue 6, September 2012, Page 454, https://doi.org/10.1093/occmed/kqs089. Copyright © The Author 2012.

Why I became an occupational physician …

Peter Verow

My medical career could be described as unorthodox and the academics at St Mary's Hospital in London did not understand my desire to have a break from medicine to play full-time squash. 'You may not be able to get back into medicine again,' they said, 'and if you do it is likely that you will only have the option to become a GP!' I followed my own instincts and after house jobs became a 'full-time squash player'. I have never regretted the career break, travelling around the world and learning the need to win to survive.

Eventually all good things come to an end, and having recognized that a sports career is short and not very lucrative, I had to return to medicine after a few years. My re-entry was provided through contacts and a shortage of anaesthetists and after a phone call from somewhere deep in Mexico I became an anaesthetic senior house officer (SHO) in Birmingham. A series of other SHO posts enabled me to complete my general practitioner vocational training programme and I began somewhat half-heartedly looking for a full-time partnership. By chance, I noticed an advertisement for a trainee occupational physician with the Rover Car group in Birmingham and, by coincidence, Nick Trethowan who was working at the Institute of Occupational Medicine and living quite close was able to tell me more about the speciality and convinced me that it was worth a try.

Longbridge was an ideal place to gain one's first experience of occupational medicine. There was plenty of onsite medical emergencies as well as experience of confrontation during the era of union power and 'Red Robbo'. Ian Picton-Robinson, my trainer, encouraged me to visit other sites to learn more about the different aspects of the speciality. Having completed 2 years of Membership of the Faculty of Occupational Medicine (MFOM) training, Ian helped me to persuade the powers to be that I could undertake my final 2 years MFOM training within a new National Health Service (NHS) post at Sandwell, where I have remained ever since. Ironically, despite all the advice of those St Mary's academics, I have now ended up an NHS hospital consultant. While it has taken some time to educate them about what occupational physicians actually do, the opportunity to work closely with other consultants has led to a greater respect for each other's' roles and needs.

NHS occupational medicine has enabled me to work regular hours, participate in teaching and research and provide a better working environment for NHS employees. My study leave even allowed me to attend an 'Olympic Games' as the medical officer to the Great Britain gold medal-winning hockey team to complete my MFOM dissertation. I do not think that would be allowed today!

I have no regrets that by chance I found occupational medicine. Perhaps the new F1/F2 training years for junior doctors will provide more opportunities to raise the awareness of our speciality and thereby leave less to chance in the future.

Source: *Occupational Medicine*, Volume 56, Issue 6, September 2006, Page 429, https://doi.org/10.1093/occmed/kql032. Copyright © The Author 2006.

Fifty years ago:
'The Diseases of Occupations by Donald Hunter'

L.G. Norman

It is fortunate for medical men and women who give their services to industry that one of the finest teachers of medicine should have devoted so much of his life's work to the study of the influence of occupations upon disease. This fascinating subject attracts the attention of many physicians in a sporadic manner, but in the past 120 years or so only four general physicians have published major works on it. Donald Hunter takes his place beside Thackrah (1832), Arlidge (1892), Oliver (1908) and Legge (1934); indeed, with the accumulated knowledge of the present generation, he leads them all.

This book should prove a valuable stimulus to the teaching of occupational health, of great help to both students and teachers. Neither it is a reference work for Industrial Medical Officers on points of detail nor is it intended as such; it will however be invaluable for any medical man or woman who is taking up an industrial appointment for the first time. The text is refreshingly free from typographical errors. There are >400 excellent photographs which in themselves form a useful education in industrial processes and illustrate many occupational diseases. There are >1000 references which cover each subject well as a guide to more detailed reading.

Dr Hunter has amply fulfilled his purpose of reviewing 'on a broad basis and with emphasis on its clinical aspects the problem of disease, in relation to occupation'. This book will be our guide for many years in teaching and in encouraging our colleagues in other branches of medicine to develop an interest and perhaps even an enthusiasm for the study of the diseases of occupations. It does not matter if the details of our own special concern are sometimes not set out as fully as we should wish; what matters is that occupational health in general will gain in stature by the publication of this work by one of the leading consultant physicians of our day.

Source: *Occupational Medicine*, Volume 56, Issue 8, December 2006, Page 520, https://doi.org/10.1093/occmed/kql128. Copyright © The Author 2006.

Originally from: *Occup Med (Lond)*1956;6.

Health and safety legislation

Mike Gibson

Early legislation on health and safety exists dating back to mediaeval times, for example the Textus Roffensis or Aethelbehrt's code, but this tended to be retributional, setting punishment for direct physical attack along biblical lines or 'an eye for an eye'. Modern health and safety legislation really started in the United Kingdom with the Factories Act in 1833, which was expanded by other Acts of Parliament relating to particular industries, such as mining and quarrying. The first, overarching legislation was the Health & Safety at Work Act in 1974. This in turn was expanded by secondary legislation of which the 'Six Pack' is an example. More recently, the law has been tidied by further legislation. However, the 9th Abbot of Iona, Adomnán mac Rónáin, drafted a law that predates the 1974 Act by almost 1400 years. Meyer [1] translated the Lex Innocentium, or the Law of Adomnán, which was adopted at the Synod of Birr in Co. Offaly in 697 AD. It was unusual in being written in Old Irish. Grigg suggests [2] that this shows it was a law for the people, as other law was written in Latin. Lex Innocentium was primarily concerned with the protection from attack of women, children and the clergy, but Clancy and Crawford [3] claim that the following extract

> For every woman that has been slain, whether a man has a share in it ... for everything that is made liable under the Law, both ditch and pit and bridge and hearth and doorstep and pools and kilns and every other harm besides

demonstrates provision for partial culpability for industrial accidents and dangerous workmanship. It was the concept of recompense for damage to the individual caused indirectly that was unusual. The Law also made liable those who offended through ignorance, neglect or lack of intervention. Although the Law was guaranteed by over 100 bishops, other clerics and kings of Ireland, Pictland and Dalriada, no evidence of cases brought under the Law survives—although O'Donovan et al. [4] quote examples of punishment for homicide, which appear to be in accordance with the Law.

References

1. **Meyer K.** *Cáin Adomnain: An Old Irish Treatise on the Law of Adomnán.* Oxford: Clarendon Press, 1905.
2. **Grigg J.** Aspects of the Cáin: Adomnán's Lex Innocentium. *J Aust Early Medieval Assoc* 2005;1:41–50.
3. **Clancy TO, Crawford BE.** The formation of the Scottish Kingdom, p. 116. In: Houston RA, Knox WWJ, eds. *The History of Scotland.* London: The Folio Society, 2006.
4. **O'Donovan J,** ed. *Annals of the Kings of Ireland by the Four Masters, Vol. 2 at M907.6.* Dublin: Hodges, Smith & Co., 1856.

Source: *Occupational Medicine,* Volume 64, Issue 6, September 2014, Page 441, https://doi.org/10.1093/occmed/kqu084. Copyright © The Author 2014.

How one pre-employment decision nearly changed the world order

Nerys Williams

Asthmatic from the age of 2, our subject was unable to attend school and had to be educated at home. As a teenager, he was found unfit for military service and so studied medicine. He qualified after only 3 years and became interested in allergies, presenting his work at conferences and publishing papers in the Journal of Allergy.

During his extended 'gap' year, he worked as a stevedore, porter, dishwasher and in a leper colony. He became concerned about the malnutrition, poverty and misery and wrote about the role of the doctor. He gathered statistics and wrote about the lack of state protection and health care for poor people.

A meeting with a charismatic lawyer changed his focus in life and he became an expedition doctor for a group of revolutionaries who shared his ideal of improving the lot of the poor. They became intent on the overthrow of a corrupt regime.

The invasion by sea did not go well with only 12 surviving from an initial army of 82. He had forgotten his asthma medication and was severely debilitated by one of his frequent attacks during the crossing. He injected adrenaline to combat symptoms and within weeks of landing and entering jungle, he made a life-changing decision—he put down his medicine bag, took up a gun and became not the 'doctor' but a fighter. He became an expert in guerrilla warfare and wrote the definitive book on the subject. He used his antiasthma vaporizer to aspirate rainwater from puddles in the jungle and provided water for the men to drink.

Skirmishes with the military led to several injuries but none more embarrassing than when his pistol fell to the floor and fired, hitting him on the cheek. Fetid jungle conditions aggravated his asthma as did the lint hammock and he was given special permission to use one made from canvas.

He did not totally dispense with being a doctor—he set up clinics in villages and saw cases of rickets, parasitism and avitaminosis—the experience confirmed his view that only political change would improve the plight of the poor.

Against the odds, the revolutionaries succeeded and he became head of the national bank in the new government. He developed the moon face of steroid dependency but continued to smoke large cigars. He tried acupuncture for his asthma while on a visit to China. It failed to provide relief.

Disillusionment with the new order set in and he set off on his travels again trying to export the concept of a fairer society. Ultimately, he met his fate at the hands of the USA who greatly feared his views and intentions.

His face remains iconic yet few people remember he was a doctor, had extensive knowledge of workers and a clear but violent strategy to improve their lives. Had Che Guevara been passed as fit for military service, the world really might have been a different place and students would have to find someone else to adorn their walls.

Source: *Occupational Medicine*, Volume 58, Issue 7, October 2008, Page 519, https://doi.org/10.1093/occmed/kqn095. Copyright © The Author 2008.

Reprinted by permission of Oxford University Press on behalf of the Society of Occupational Medicine.

Why I became an occupational physician ...

Susan A. Robson

My reaction on being asked to write about 'Why I became an occupational physician' was astonishment that anyone could be interested in my career, followed by a degree of despondency as it felt as if I was being asked to write my own obituary. I asked myself—am I really that old?! Like many other contributors, I can sum up the reasons in two words and those are 'fortunate chance'. Looking back has made me realize the significant changes in society and medicine during my 37-year career. I came from a very rural area where it was somewhat uncommon for women to study medicine and if married with children, at the very most you would only work part time.

I was fortunate to go to King's College, Durham (subsequently the University of Newcastle) with a Department of Industrial Medicine. Undergraduate teaching from Richard Browne and Ian McCallum kindled an interest in the subject reinforced by romantic involvement with an engineering student who also attended the same lectures.

After qualification, I married that same engineering student and entered general practice as this enabled me to continue working while following my husband to various Unilever businesses around the country. At that time, large organizations held the paternalistic view that the wife would always follow the husband! Sleepless nights worrying how I could continue my career following a proposed move to South Africa were unfounded as we were posted instead to St Andrews where I had a mixed portfolio of work in General Practice, Family Planning and in the University Health Service with Inglis Lamont. As a student, I had known Stan Pomford, the Director of the East of Scotland Occupational Health Service and he asked me to provide some help. I immediately took to the variety of activities involved with what was emerging as a new speciality. I vividly remember my 'light on the road to Damascus' (in my case the Tay Bridge!) when my husband suggested that I should look to developing my own career. Fortunately, there was a full-time course in Industrial Medicine at the University of Dundee and I joined an excellent group of students including Eric Teasdale and Alan Reid. Following the next move to Chester, I was approached by Ken Lee, the County Medical Adviser for Cheshire and one of the founder members of ALAMA. He proved an exceptional mentor and encouraged me to complete my dissertation and to take over his post when he retired. You could say that the rest is history!!

I have lived through an exciting time with the development of the speciality and in common with many of my illustrious colleagues I have never regretted my move into occupational medicine. It has proved a tailor-made job for me and I have very much enjoyed my career. I am fortunate indeed that I was in the right place at the right time and met exceptional individuals who encouraged me to take advantage of all the opportunities available.

Source: *Occupational Medicine*, Volume 56, Issue 7, October 2006, Page 441, https://doi.org/10.1093/occmed/kql065. Copyright © The Author 2006.

DDA 1995, 2005 or 605?

Hanaa Sayed

The Disability Discrimination Act 1995 (DDA, 1995) (amended 2005) aims to prevent discrimination against people with disabilities at work. It is interesting to note that >1400 years ago a very similar principle applied. The Arabs who embraced Islam had five pillars to follow; three of them are DDA compliant. The first two 'pillars' are to do with certain beliefs and to give charity (as a percentage of their savings) where the DDA does not apply!

The third pillar is praying which is done five times a day and involves standing and bending. People with disabilities are entitled to adjustments such as praying while sitting down to avoid the bending. Very unwell people can even pray while lying down flat!

The next pillar is fasting where one does not eat or drink from sunrise to sunset. People with certain medical conditions (for example diabetics) are exempt from fasting altogether and are asked to feed the poor instead. Healthy ladies who are pregnant or breastfeeding are also entitled to the same adjustment.

The fifth one is Hajj (pilgrimage) which involves walking for miles. People with disabilities are allowed to do it on a wheelchair or may be exempted altogether according to their disability.

Age is also carefully considered. Children (defined as pre-puberty) are exempted from fasting and pilgrimage. The elderly are defined by being too old and unwell rather than by age. They are exempt from pilgrimage and fasting.

Another 'ancient ritual' is infection control. For >1400 years, Muslims believe they should eat or drink using only the right hand. They can use only the left hand for personal hygiene in the toilet.

Source: *Occupational Medicine*, Volume 57, Issue 8, December 2007, Page 617, https://doi.org/10.1093/occmed/kqm101. Copyright © The Author 2007.

Reprinted by permission of Oxford University Press on behalf of the Society of Occupational Medicine.

Fifty years ago: 'The work of the Research Advisory Committee'

D. Malcolm

Given at a meeting of the Association on 3 April 1964 by D. Malcolm, Chief Medical Officer Chloride Electrical Storage Company Limited.

The criticism has been made that the Research *Advisory* Committee does not carry out much research—I have made it myself in the past. However, it is obvious that a committee meeting four to six times a year cannot itself undertake research and its title is 'The Research Advisory Committee'. At the first meeting, Dr Glover suggested that the Committee might take a more active part in stimulating and coordinating research amongst Association members. Previous committees had discussed this on several occasions and had been aware of the difficulties. Perhaps, the most important change is the replacement of the word 'help' by 'promote' (Table 28.1). The intention here was that the committee should actively stimulate research, rather than wait until it was asked for help.

During the past 2 years, the following subjects have been discussed: (1) A controlled trial of silicone-methyl cellulose barrier creams. (2) Investigations into occupations with known high mortality rates from bronchitis. (3) Blood pressure estimations amongst lead workers. (4) This year, the committee plans to hold a research symposium on the subject of cadmium, to see if certain practical questions can be answered. (5) The commissioning of authoritative articles on practical subjects of interest to doctors in industry. These articles would be written by experts in their subject and printed from time to time in *The Transactions*.

From what has been said, it should be obvious that neither the committee nor the majority of members of the Association are able to engage in full-time research. Nevertheless, there are many problems requiring answers in the wide field covered by occupational medicine. Many members must have problems in common to which they would like a clear answer, and such an answer might be found by pooling all their experience. As an example, some time ago the committee was asked to give evidence to the Committee on Prescribed Diseases on the effect of acid spray on the teeth. Work on this subject had been published, but the number of cases was limited.

Table 28.1. Old and new terms of reference

Old terms of reference	New terms of reference
1 To help members of the Association with research.	1 To promote the interest of members in Occupational Health research.
2 To initiate research projects.	2 To act as a link between Industrial Medical Officers and recognized research bodies.
3 To make funds available for research, where projects were felt to be worthy of support and the support was of the kind that could be given by the Association.	3 To initiate research within the Association.
	4 To consider methods of helping members who wish to undertake their own research.

Some authorities even said that acid did not affect the teeth. At this time, I was co-opted to the Research Advisory Committee and asked to give evidence. We received a great deal of help from the committee in getting this evidence out in suitable statistical form and it was later suggested that it should be published in the *British Journal of Industrial Medicine*. Many of us have carried out investigations to provide practical answers to our own problems. Such 'knowhow', which one can never find in the textbooks or 'scientific' literature, is only slowly passed around—if you know whom to ask. Surely, much of this work is worth publishing and our own *Transactions* would seem to be the right place to publish it.

Source: *Occupational Medicine*, Volume 64, Issue 3, April 2014, Page 228, https://doi.org/10.1093/occmed/kqu029. Copyright © The Author 2014.

Originally from: The work of the Research Advisory Committee. *Trans Ass Industr Med Offrs* (1964) 14:56. Available at: *Occup Med (Lond)* 1964;14:56–58. DOI:10.1093/ occmed/14.1.56.

I want never gets

Anthony Seaton

'I want it!'—perhaps the first sentence we use as infants. The well brought up child soon learns the automatic parental response—'I want never gets; say "Please may I have?"'

The verb 'to want' reflects a basic need of all living organisms described by the noun 'want', derived from the Old Norse, *vanta* or lack. For many people, want of the fundamental necessities of life, water, food and family support is a reality. As children in the 1940s, we were admonished to eat up and remember the starving children in China; even then we were well off compared with most of the world's people. Our parents provided us with other things that indicated that the world surrounding us was rich in treasures there for the asking. 'I want' became a test of the extent of this provision; to want had become to covet (Old French, *coveitier* from Latin, *cupiditas*, desire or longing).

I see this change occurring in my grandchildren around the age of 6 months, as they explore the world around them. Reflex grasping and turning towards the mother's breast is transferred to other new and interesting objects that are tested for taste and feel. Many children now have a full set of grandparents who can be trained to provide further delights. How unsurprising that by the time Mrs Thatcher came to power a generation was conditioned to expect more than their parents had ever dreamed of. To covet had become acceptable; to some, even greed was good.

Perhaps this conversion of want to covet is hard-wired into us. However, like most genetic determinants, it can be modified by our environment, as recognized in all faiths. Nevertheless, covetousness is the primary motivation of capitalism, leading to competition for resources. For the last 250 years, the world's economy has been driven by this basic urge. In Adam Smith's time, resources of water, iron and coal were unlimited and the possibility of increasing national prosperity was obvious. Malthus pointed to the dangers of overpopulation but agriculture kept pace and the population of these islands increased, although shortages still brought episodic starvation. The West led the world in economic growth and exploitation of the world's resources. Having plundered the world to satisfy our own covetousness, we cannot be surprised that less favoured nations aspire to emulate us. But now, we know that resources are not infinite and our capacity to absorb waste is close to saturation. The lesson taught by Malthus has not been heeded and the world's population has reached the point at which its needs for energy and food are unlikely to be satisfied. Covetousness is being replaced again by want.

Can we restrict freedom to reproduce and to plunder the Earth while entering into international agreements to decelerate economic growth? History suggests that we cannot but that nature will do it for us. Want of water, food and energy with accompanying war and plagues were known to the ancient Egyptians and the Israelites and ever since then have determined the course of the tribes of mankind. Now these wants are global.

Source: *Occupational Medicine*, Volume 59, Issue 2, March 2009, Page 132, https://doi.org/10.1093/occmed/kqn118. Copyright © The Author 2009.

Why I became an occupational physician …

David Wright

Occupational medicine is rarely a first choice career for those entering medicine and it probably should not be. A wider training in other specialities gives the occupational physician an understanding of illnesses, ailments and patients and in contrast to many other branches of medicine, it is the response to illness or adversity rather than the illness itself that is important.

Having dallied with surgery following qualification, I decided it was not for me. I had no real view of what I should do and decided that a short service commission in the Army would at least give me time to reach some sort of conclusion. Somewhat unusually, I joined the Royal Scots Dragoon Guards directly under the regimental doctor scheme, initially for 3 years. The first couple of years were in Germany, essentially in general practice. This was not for me either! What was of real interest was the health needs of the soldier in barracks, in the field and on operations. Although I did not realize it at the time, occupational medicine is never more real than when the doctor lives in sometimes very uncomfortable and unpleasant circumstances along with those he supports. A very full understanding of the issues develops with a commitment to do something positive about them.

Short service extended into long service. Attendance at the Staff College delayed higher professional training but did help crystallize my views. In the services, there is considerable overlap between occupational and public health medicine, many posts combining aspects of the two. At the time of the formation of the two faculties, the general view in the services was that community medicine (as it was known at the time) would be the preferred option. During my time in posts following staff training, it became clear in my own mind that occupational medicine was the right way to go.

Formal training started with the Occupational Medicine MSc course at the London School of Hygiene and Tropical Medicine. Unfortunately, the decision was then made to close the department and this inevitably had its effects. Nevertheless, there were those committed few who continued to ensure that effective training was given. Higher professional training continued in a variety of posts in the services including a spell in the Devonport Dockyard. Before completing this, I was whisked away to be the Chief Medical Officer of the United Nations Protection Force in Yugoslavia. I was still trying to complete my Membership of the Faculty of Occupational Medicine dissertation faxing revised submissions over a satellite link from a war torn Sarajevo which can help put other aspects of working life in perspective at times.

Would I take the same path again? Certainly. Occupational medicine completes the medical process and rather than treating a disease or illness *per se* it looks at the whole person and their response. Instead of having discharge from hospital or clinic as the end point of intervention, occupational physicians have the very real target of a return to a productive life.

Source: *Occupational Medicine*, Volume 56, Issue 8, December 2006, Page 583, https://doi.org/10.1093/occmed/kql067. Copyright © The Author 2006.

Reprinted by permission of Oxford University Press on behalf of the Society of Occupational Medicine.

Why I became a second hand bookseller: part 1

Andy Slovak

'It's nice work if you can get it, sitting behind that desk and taking in money for all this rubbish; I wish I could do it.'

'Yes madam, once you've trained the replacement stock to jump up onto the shelves and all the books to retidy themselves at the end of the day; there's nothing to it.'

Sue and I got into the book trade by having 'interests', which needed feeding by the acquisition of out-of-print books. In my case, the original one was the representation of war in children's fiction during the first half of the 20th century. I took to haunting auction rooms and, as most books are sold in multi-box lots, I soon acquired a stock. My first salutary lesson was that putting the stuff back into auction was a dead loss. My second happier lesson was that going to the odd fair or history event and selling them was fun and subsidized the collecting. Thus, a dealer was born.

Also at that time, the early to mid-1980s, it was still possible to go to 'Hay on Weigh' and buy books by the kilogram and fill the car for a few hundred pounds. Provided that one could find one or two niches to specialize in (mine are radical history and science), then one could do comfortably well at the fairs and I also started putting stock into chums' bookshops. (People will often not go upstairs for new books but the lure of rooting about for junk often draws them: particularly husbands.)

The catalysts for getting into the business more seriously were stopping full-time work in 2003, the closure of a couple of my friends' operations and the sudden and urgent offer of a huge number of books from a public school. They had been told on inspection that they were not a book museum and that they could not shelve books above six feet rather than the then eighteen. For several years afterwards, the school librarian was rung by crusty old gentlemen to tell him that some rascally Norfolk book dealer was flogging off his tomes. His replies got terser and terser with time.

The first problem was a venue. Location, as we are told by the TV pundits, is all. The thing with books is that once they have been seen by the local population of collectors and enthusiasts, they are, for all practical intents and purposes, dead stock. One either turns them over or one turns over the clientele. The latter being easier on my back, we started to hunt for premises in a holiday venue. Sue having strong family connections to North Norfolk, we began there. She spotted a property for auction on a Wednesday, bought on Friday and blocked drains and dry rot discovered on Saturday. But it was on the main street and in a good spot near the church and museum. A mere 2 years of building work later, we were ready to open our shop, Much Binding.

Source: *Occupational Medicine*, Volume 60, Issue 4, June 2010, Page 321, https://doi.org/10.1093/occmed/kqq015. Copyright © The Author 2010.

Tales of Kieran: The occupational physician's odyssey 2—New job

J.A. Hunter

Kieran, my Occupational Physician friend, has answered the call from academia, and whilst Linbridge is more a city of steaming piles than dreaming spires, in common parlance, 'the boy done well'. After five years at Lincaster Health Authority he has certainly made his mark, and after I saw his old job advertised I decided to give him a ring.

Kieran sounded like the proverbial cat with cream; it was a new post, he was to become a fellow of St Arrhenius College and he even had full access to the College croquet lawn. What's more, old Prof. Hailstone had put his arm around him and suggested that Kieran might like to contribute to the next edition of Closet's *Compleat Textbook of Medicine*.

But how would Lincaster fill the black hole that Kieran's departure would leave?

'Well of course, this is a major and established post now,' he boomed down the telephone, 'and we have high hopes of attracting a quality candidate to continue the kind of work we have produced here.' Indeed, the advert had been one of those full-page glossy affairs that demands attention and sought 'applications from established Occupational Physicians with full accreditation'.

So had the lines been buzzing with interest?

'Well no, not exactly, apart from a few local GPs, and I made it perfectly plain to them that at the very least they must have the full MFOM.' And that was telling them.

I dropped in to the Department a fortnight later to find Kieran practising academic poses presumably for his acceptance speech. 'Any interest on the replacement front?' I inquired and immediately detected the smell of cream turning sour. 'One' came the reply eventually reflected off the mirror, 'but he does look quite interesting. Take a look at the CV.' Jeanne, his secretary, looked decidedly nervous as she handed it to me and then hastily departed from the room.

It did look quite good as I flicked through; trained in the Steel Industry before work in the South American mining industry and then Health and Safety Executive, not too dissimilar from Kieran himself, I thought to myself. It was only when I read the references from Professor Eggon D. Phace and Dr Bart Simpson that I started to smell a rat.

I managed to corner Jeanne before I left. She told me how disappointed he had been when nobody applied so she and the Ocupational Health nurse spent a whole afternoon concocting an application thinking he would surely see through Professor Eggon D. Phace. But no, he was so impressed that he had arranged an interview date with Personnel and the Appointments Committee as soon as he finished reading it. The poor woman looked quite distraught and just couldn't understand why Kieran had not twigged. 'Why' she said 'it's his own CV!'

As they say, the surest form of flattery …

Source: *Occupational Medicine*, Volume 52, Issue 3, 1 May 2002, Page 167, https://doi.org/10.1093/occmed/52.3.167. Copyright © Society of Occupational Medicine 2002.

Reprinted with permission from Hunter J. A. (1991) *Lancet*, 338(8773):1009.

The oldest sick note

John Hobson

A 450-year-old letter written by Mary Queen of Scots excusing a nobleman from his duties was sold at auction earlier this year for £6000 [1]. Dated 14 March 1554 it has been described as the world's oldest sick note and was sent by Mary to the Laird of Blair, relieving him of his duties at court as he was suffering from gout. Gout, traditionally an affliction of the rich, was even worn as a badge of honour rather than the more common rheumatism. Many famous individuals have suffered from gout including Martin Luther, Sir Isaac Newton and Thomas Jefferson. But in the bicentennial year of his birth, England's greatest fictional author not only suffered with the condition but featured it repeatedly in his writing. Sam Weller, in the *Pickwick Papers*, cautions his father against excessive drinking fearing it will bring the old man another attack. In *Bleak House*, Sir Leicester Dedlock is resigned to his fate as a sufferer of the family gout, passed down through the generations. He describes it as his 'old faithful ally' which 'grips him by both legs'. The suffering of these characters preceded the onset of Dickens's own gout in his left foot at the age of 52. It plagued him in the last years of his life, had a deleterious effect on his lifestyle [2] and may have been partially responsible for the significant reduction in his literary output during this time. The associated metabolic syndrome probably contributed to his death six years later from a stroke. Dickens was a famous reformer and campaigned for the improvement of social conditions. He had experience of working in a blacking factory, putting soot into pots and drew on this experience for his writing. He visited the mills in Manchester to see and report on the working conditions there.

Gout is the most common form of inflammatory arthritis in men over the age of 40 with an estimated prevalence in the UK of 1.4% [3]. Over 60% of sufferers have metabolic syndrome and have a higher risk of death mainly because of vascular disease. The incidence and prevalence of gout has markedly increased over the last few decades and its association with alcohol, dietary purines and fructose ingestion has been confirmed and explains why it was formerly seen as a disease of the affluent. New treatments have been developed including interleukin-1 antagonists for acute gout and febuxostat and pegloticase for chronic gout. Vitamin C supplements reduce the risk of gout.

'A sovereign cure for the gout' said Mr Pickwick hastily producing his notebook 'What is it?' 'The gout sir,' replied Mr Weller 'the gout is a complaint as arises from too much ease and comfort. If ever you're attacked with the gout, sir, jist you marry a widder as has got a good loud woice, with a decent notion of usin' it, and you'll never have the gout agin....I can warrant it to drive away any illness as is caused by too much jollity.' [4].

References

1. BBC News 8 March 2012. www.bbc.co.uk/news.
2. Tomalin C. *Charles Dickens: A Life*. Penguin, 2012.
3. Suresh E, Das P. Recent advances in management of gout. *Q J Med* 2012;**105**:407–417.
4. Dickens C. *The Posthumous Papers of the Pickwick Club*. Public Domain Books, 2006.

Source: *Occupational Medicine*, Volume 62, Issue 7, October 2012, Page 518, https://doi.org/10.1093/occmed/kqs120. Copyright © The Author 2012.

Reprinted by permission of Oxford University Press on behalf of the Society of Occupational Medicine.

Why I became an occupational physician …

Joseph L. Kearns

In gratitude for their prompt help in a serious accident in a new sewer tunnel outside the Norfolk and Norwich Hospital, the medical staff were invited to see the work excavating the wide bore, using as a rough guide the layer of pebbles on what had been the bed of the Rhine 18 000 years ago. That was so interesting that registrars arranged visits to other local enterprises, including Colman's mustard factory. Our curiosity was such that at the West Norwich Hospital, during a polio epidemic, everyone in the mess took a turn inside an iron lung, the better to understand how to brief a distressed, breathless patient on what to expect when incarcerated helplessly within a controlled environment.

During my own National Service in the RAMC, I had to assess and maintain the fitness of 120 recruits arriving every fortnight as they performed a wide variety of tasks. Later, I did the same to Civil Service candidates and sickness absentees in the London postal district of W12.

At the end of a weekly session for general practitioners at the Hammersmith Hospital, a participant asked those assembled, 'Would anybody like to look after Cadby Hall during my holidays?' Mine was the only response. Bill Blood had been an architect of the Diploma in Industrial Health, and informally introduced me to the specialism as I cared for 8500 employees of J. Lyons and Company for 3 weeks each year. On one occasion, my boss Sir Samuel Salmon attended me with a sore foot. I asked him to lean on the examination couch while I raised the sole of his foot behind him. Cigar ablaze, he exclaimed over his shoulder 'You're treating a knight of the Realm like a bloody horse!'.

Five years later Bill fell terminally ill. Sir Samuel would not contemplate him reading of his replacement as he lay dying, so he asked me to remain until Bill died. I was then offered the opportunity to study while my locum was paid. I could have the job if I gained the DIH. My wife and Stuart Carne, my partners in general practice, encouraged me to try. If I failed or did not like the career change, I would always be welcome back.

At SOM meetings, Bill had not been allowed to speak unless he introduced himself as 'Blood, of Lyons!' Mere 'Kearns', having burned no bridges, was incredibly lucky to be introduced to a new career, mentored by Jackie O'Dwyer of Unilever, Jimmy Grahame of Heinz, Andrew Raffle of London Transport and Roy Archibald of the National Coal Board. Lyons later encouraged me to host meetings with John Aldridge of IBM, Roger Treadgold of UCH, Harold Bridger and Alexis Brook of the Tavistock Institute and several other senior colleagues, to consider how we might help our managements to understand, assess and control the total working environment.

My apparently aimless wanderings have proved to be an exciting, fulfilling progression full circle!

Source: *Occupational Medicine*, Volume 57, Issue 1, January 2007, Page 74, https://doi.org/10.1093/occmed/kql070. Copyright © The Author 2006.

Why I became a second hand bookseller: part 2

Andy Slovak

The rules of the game are quite simple but they have to be stuck to. If you do, and are lucky, then you can survive and modestly prosper. If you do not, then the Swanee awaits. We do have a business plan. It is written on the back of a small cornflakes packet. But we do stick to it, and it works. The key issue is price of purchase of stock. It must reflect the certainty that only a proportion (~20 to 30%) will be sold at profit. So, if you have offered stuff to a few local dealers yourself and have been suspicious when they have all offered you much the same (disappointing?) price, be reassured. It is not a conspiracy: they are all just working to the same rules of survival. (There are some rascals too, but surprisingly few.)

The joy of books lies in their aesthetics, the feel of fine cloth paper, the fragility of wartime ephemera, the beauties of some long neglected illustrator and the discovery of previously unknown or forgotten writers of great power but the true joys of dealing are in the customers.

We have discovered that a fat man with a rucksack has the same 'footprint' as a wheelchair and that a fat couple can effectively 'kettle' half a coach load of customers. The noisily appreciative middle classes seldom buy anything, whereas the EYMs (Earnest Young Men) quietly hoover up a stack of books and appear suddenly and shyly happy with their haul at our desk. In the high summer, we have much Driftwood (drift in: drift out: thick as planks) also known as Brownians (from the motion of the same name).

Couples are fascinating. There is quite a broad spectrum of nerdal preoccupation in our clientele and the tolerance and encouragement of the other partner, when present, is very sweet. The opposite phenomenon, of contemptuous or harsh intolerance, is sadly commoner; usually in the female partner. We call them BMWs (Bottom Mouthed Women) from the shape of distaste that their mouths assume (Oh no, not another bookshop!).

Male customers, on their own, often declaim their needs in simple statements without preamble or by your leave, thus 'Traction engines' or 'Hogarth' or 'Exotic photography'. Our favourite was a chap who walked in and announced 'Rigid PVC pipework'. 'Yes sir, do you know the author and ISBN number?' After a little more gentle ribbing, we sent him over the road to the hardware shop where we assume his needs were satisfied.

For those interested, a collection of remarks overheard in bookshops was made under the title of *Bookworm's Droppings* by Shaun Tyas.

It is well worth looking for.

As doctors, we are somewhat insulated by behavioural norms from the awfulness, condescension and tedium of a proportion of humankind but probably also from much spontaneity and delight from discovering among our stock both long lost friends and new joys. So far, it has been fun and we are now going into our fifth year.

Source: *Occupational Medicine*, Volume 60, Issue 6, September 2010, Page 495, https://doi.org/10.1093/occmed/kqq016. Copyright © The Author 2010.

Fifty years ago: 'The first group occupational health service in Scotland'

W.M. Dixon

Given at the Annual Provincial Meeting on 15 July 1964.

Development of group occupational health services in Britain, at least in modern times, began in 1947 with Slough and was followed in 1955 by Harlow (Taylor, 1959) and later by Dr Garland's service around the Central Middlesex Hospital. Dundee, Rochdale and Smethwick thus represent the second generation of such services founded with the help of the Nuffield Foundation.

In July 1960, it was announced by the Minister of Labour in the House of Commons that £250 000 had been set aside by the Nuffield Foundation, largely to encourage the formation of such services in old, established industrial areas. Professor A. Mair of the University of St Andrews felt that Dundee would be a suitable place for such a venture. He and the District Factory Inspector, Mr T. Graham, worked hard for many months to drum up enthusiasm for the scheme amongst local employers, at the same time drawing the attention of the Ministry of Labour and the Nuffield Foundation to Dundee's claims. Independently, the Foundation and the Ministry of Labour had together arrived at the conclusion that Dundee would indeed be an eminently suitable choice in relation to a number of other possibilities.

Dundee is a city standing on the north shore of the River Tay in the east of Scotland, about halfway between Edinburgh and Aberdeen. With a population of 190 000, it is Scotland's third largest city, but the second in industrial importance. Of the insured working population of 90 000 some 18 000 are jute workers. The remainder work in a wide variety of industries, some of which are housed in new factory buildings on industrial estates on the outskirts of the city. The rest are in older factories, some of which have been modernized, but many remain as they were before the war.

Efforts to promote an industrial health service in Dundee suffered many setbacks but finally in the spring of 1962, these were successful. A group of 14 employers agreed to the formation of a service, but their employees totalled only 3500. The Nuffield Foundation felt that unless 5000 people were forthcoming, it would be unwise to begin. At that time the University in Dundee was looking for a new Student Health Officer, as their existing arrangements were only temporary. When Queen's College agreed to join the Service, the minimum of 5000, which the Nuffield Foundation felt to be essential, was reached. Amongst the founders, therefore, there was a unique one in the shape of the University itself.

The founder members formed a limited liability non-profit-making company, and a Council of Management was elected. The Council is composed of 10 members elected from those firms who founded the service. A third will retire in October and be replaced by election each year. An equal number of Council members are invited from organizations representative of the Dundee business community, the trade unions, the National Health Service, the University and the Nuffield Foundation.

Source: *Occupational Medicine*, Volume 64, Issue 4, June 2014, Page 293, https://doi.org/10.1093/occmed/kqu030. Copyright © The Author 2014.

Originally from: The first group occupational health service in Scotland. *Trans Ass Industr Med Offrs* (1964) 14, 66. Available at: *Occupational Medicine*, Volume 14, Issue 1, 1 April 1964, Pages 66–72.

I learned (a bit) about aviation medicine from that

Mike Gibson

Over 40 years ago, I was a very new, junior medical officer at an RAF flying training school. On one morning surgery day, I was asked by one of the pilots and his wife to arrange for him to undergo a vasectomy. As an Aberdeen graduate, I was used to stoic farmers from the Mearns. On one occasion, when I was doing sperm counts in surgical outpatients in Aberdeen, one such stalwart had commented to me that he did not think his vasectomy had worked. He explained that when he did it to his bullocks, their testicles had swollen and fallen off—and his had not. I also had in mind the vision of a Royal Naval doctor of my acquaintance who had his vasectomy performed under local anaesthetic, after which he cycled back to work.

I briefed our intrepid pilot on what was involved and how the operation was done and I arranged for the local Simon Clinic to carry out the procedure, as neither the NHS nor the RAF offered the service in our region. He had the operation and, unknown to me, returned to flying the next day. After his first sortie, he was brought to the station medical centre by an admiring group of colleagues. He was virtually unable to walk as a result of a scrotal haematoma about the size of an ostrich egg. I had obviously not reminded him to avoid activities that could induce complications such as haematoma. It transpired that his sortie had involved aerobatics and the pulling of up to 5g.

Allowing a central venous pressure of 5 mmHg and a measurement from the right atrium to the scrotum of 17 inches, the normal orthostatic pressure at the level of the scrotum would be in the order of 36 mmHg. The level of centrifugal force involved would therefore have exerted approximately 180 mmHg of venous pressure at the site of surgery. Fortunately, he was able to pass urine without difficulty and the condition resolved in a few days with mild analgesia and the use of a jock strap—and abstinence from flying. But I did learn a bit about aviation medicine from that ... and it did cost me a few pints of beer.

Source: *Occupational Medicine*, Volume 64, Issue 7, October 2014, Page 545, https://doi.org/10.1093/occmed/kqu085. Copyright © The Author 2014.

Reprinted by permission of Oxford University Press on behalf of the Society of Occupational Medicine.

Why I became an occupational physician …

Raymond Agius

The more I think about it, the more I feel that the answer to this question dates back to way before I knew what 'occupational medicine' meant. At school, I enjoyed and excelled in the sciences, especially chemistry and physics. I set up a laboratory in the basement at home and used to carry out experiments with chemicals I bought from pharmacies or fireworks factories. (I found the contents of 'chemistry sets' to be relatively innocuous and unchallenging.) Very naively I endeavoured to have available as many 'antidotes' to my chemical collection as I could muster.

In my last year of secondary school, I decided to read medicine, although at that stage I was more fascinated by 'cure' than by 'prevention'. I considered medicine to be a science (albeit very applied) rather than an art. When I started medical school, I was disappointed at how much anatomy and how relatively little chemistry featured in my preclinical years. In my clinical undergraduate training, my lengthy efforts at history taking gained praise and notoriety in equal measure, as I strove to find out 'what patient had the symptoms'. Much as I enjoyed pharmacology, I was very concerned about the disproportionate efforts of the medical profession in treating inflammation or cancer, rather than in discovering and remedying the external insults which may have brought about these conditions. In the 'industrial medicine' lectures, I was taught about 'PULHEEMS' and this did not enthuse me much, but the seeds of knowledge of 'occupational disease' began to take root in my fancy.

I recognized that I was as inept with surgical instruments as with racquets, and two years after qualifying I secured the Membership of the Royal College of Physicians. Luck and serendipity played a part, since on being appointed a houseman at the Brompton Hospital in London, I was assigned to Anthony Newman Taylor's firm. I made it a point of learning as much as I could about the jobs and chemical exposure of his patients with occupational lung disease. His mentorship made me ponder about my future specialization. After a medical registrar rotation, and research on the bronchoalveolar mast cell, I took advice from Ian McCallum. He helped me recognize the potential breadth of the work of an occupational physician and identified the 'good training jobs'—where I could become competent both in the influence of health on work as well as the converse. I therefore applied for a job at the Institute of Occupational Medicine. Fortunately, as I later discovered, Anthony Seaton moved my application into the 'short-list' pile. I landed the job in which I was to learn a great deal from him. There was no computer on my desk in those days but a large sheet of blotting paper. On it, I endeavoured to draw the chemical structure of every hazardous agent that I came across in my research or in my practice as an occupational physician. I no longer have the blotting paper but I still have the habit.

Source: *Occupational Medicine*, Volume 57, Issue 1, January 2007, Page 77, https://doi.org/10.1093/occmed/kql137. Copyright © The Author 2006.

Occupational health in India

Naomi Brecker

I spent two weeks in Hyderabad, India, as guest of the Indian Institute of Public Health and generously supported by a Faculty of Occupational Medicine Mobbs Travelling Fellowship. It was a privilege to witness occupational health practice in a different country and to realize that, although we talk about significant unmet need for occupational health in the UK, the magnitude of problems facing people working in India is far greater.

India has a working age population of approximately 500 million but less than 10% of workers are covered by existing health and safety legislation. There are frequent media reports of accidents at work. During my visit, the local paper reported 12 construction workers killed when a building collapsed, two workers killed by liquid ammonia, two nurses who died of smoke inhalation following a hospital fire and a dock worker who drowned.

For the whole of India, epidemiologists have estimated an expected annual number of occupational fatalities of 36,700, with a further 18,300,000 occupational injuries and 1,850,000 occupational diseases. However, underreporting and a paucity of reliable data are widely acknowledged. In Andhra Pradesh, 99 fatal occupational accidents were reported to the state's Factory Inspectorate in 2002. If occupational fatality rates from a comparable economy (Malaysia—11 fatalities per 100,000 workers) were applied to the 385,000 workers employed by companies submitting a return under the Factories' Act, the expected number of fatalities would rise to 385. Applying the same rate to the Andhra Pradesh working age population would give a further 10-fold rise in incidence to 3,134 expected fatalities.

Access to occupational health services is nonexistent for the vast majority of workers in India. I attended the Indian Association of Occupational Health annual conference and learnt that there is little provision outside larger national and international industries, a huge shortfall in trained occupational health professionals and limited provision of specialist training. Medical services attached to workplaces concentrate on general medical diagnosis and treatment, although exemplars of excellent occupational health practice exist. The situation may change with a new national policy on safety, health and environment at work (February 2010), but whilst the document demonstrates intentions 'to ensure safe and healthy working conditions for every man and woman in the nation', the conference was told it currently lacks plans for implementation or designated resources to achieve results.

There is no standard setting body for occupational medicine in India and hence no competence-based syllabus, guidance on expected standards of practice or specialist registration. The Indian Association of Occupational Health is the only focus of professional organisation, somewhat akin to the UK's Society of Occupational Medicine.

The need for action to improve the health and safety of the working age population in India is enormous, requiring concerted national and local action. However, I think it also presents a challenge to practitioners and their representative bodies in the developed world to find ways to foster and support occupational health practice in parts of the world where accessibility is limited and where the needs are great.

Source: *Occupational Medicine*, Volume 60, Issue 7, October 2010, Page 577, https://doi.org/10.1093/occmed/kqq104. Copyright © The Author 2010.

Reprinted by permission of Oxford University Press on behalf of the Society of Occupational Medicine.

A bit like turtles

John Challenor

They don't get on. It's a dysfunctional team. Each one of them is quite brilliant in their own way. They just don't seem to get it together as a group. Does this sound familiar?

Multidisciplinary teams (MDTs) are a fact of life brought about by a requirement for many specialisms and different grades of medical people to work together for the good of an individual patient or group of patients. Why is it that so many MDTs have to grind along in chronic pain? Was the potential for friction present even before the formation of the MDT or was it a consequence of some unfortunate exothermic reaction between some perhaps more reactive members of the team?

Palpable discomfort often exists between those of same or similar background. Such a paradox causes bewilderment among other members of the team. Initial bemusement gives way to polarization. Here is potential flocculation and eventual fragmentation; an artificial group without cohesion but with an expectation of common goals.

It only takes two persons in a team to spawn a mutation with long-term consequences. The team divides. The gulf between actors and audience widens. Wise counsel hovers off stage. What was once entertaining repertory goes national. 'No wonder theirs is a dysfunctional team—those two always at loggerheads.'

Managers come and go. The aerosol of mediation is tried. 'Oh but they were always like that. It's why he left his last post and she keeps changing secretaries.' 'Really? How did they land up in our team?' 'They both had wow factor interviews backed up with phenomenal CVs. Anyway, HR said we had to appoint.'

But the foul air persists and HR has nothing to offer. They say it is a management problem and therefore local management has to sort it out. They say we have to get on with it.

Loggerhead—a foolish person.

At loggerheads—in violent dispute or disagreement.

Loggerheads—reddish brown turtles with large heads that can hold their breath under water for over three hours.

Source: *Occupational Medicine*, Volume 59, Issue 8, December 2009, Page 555, https://doi.org/10.1093/occmed/kqp149. Copyright © The Author 2009.

41

On tenterhooks

Anthony Seaton

My introduction to occupational disease was at the age of 10, when my uncle, a rough and ready Yorkshireman, took me to the woollen mill he worked for. The noise of the machinery was unbearable, yet the female operatives were apparently talking to each other. We left quickly and I asked how they could hear in that noise. 'They're all stone deaf', he said. 'They lip read.'

Forty years later at the Institute of Occupational Medicine, I was asked to consider whether wool workers suffered lung disease as a consequence of their work. The trade union thought they did but the owners were sceptical. The Health and Safety Executive wanted data on which a protective workplace dust standard might be based. Apart from occasional reports of respiratory symptoms in some dusty processes, there was little helpful in the literature, but it did seem plausible that exposure to wool dust could cause sufficient airway irritation to cause symptoms of bronchitis or asthma, so we designed a study to investigate the relations between dust exposure, symptoms and lung function.

Some things had changed in those 40 years, but the mills were still noisy. Much of the workforce spoke Urdu, requiring some ingenuity in designing and administering the questionnaire. The industry was smaller, but still divided into many different factories, some small and some large, specializing in different parts of the process, sorting and carding, back winding, dyeing, spinning and weaving. Some were very dusty and some not. A representative sample of factories was made and the workers were examined by questionnaire and lung function testing. A method of measuring personal exposure to wool dust was agreed upon and agreement by workers and management obtained. Our confidence in finding a useful result was increased somewhat early on when our senior researcher had an attack of asthma while inspecting a carding operation, but always when embarking on such research one has a hypothesis and, although the study is designed to falsify it, one rather hopes to find a positive association. So we awaited the results of the analyses [1] on tenterhooks.

On tenterhooks—a state of painful suspense or agitated expectancy (*Oxford English Dictionary*), derived from the past participle of the Latin verb *tendere*, to stretch. And there in those woollen mills, we found them, the tenterhooks, at the finishing stage of the process of weaving worsted, as the cloth was stretched out on them. What an apt metaphor for the moment of waiting for the results after all the planning, design and hard work in execution of the plan. How it brings back memories, of the start of a race, of waiting for the results of an examination or interview, of summoning up courage to propose marriage. Like fine worsted, we have all been on tenterhooks. It is part of what makes us who we are.

Reference

1. **Love RG, Smith TA, Gurr D, Soutar CA, Scarisbrick DA, Seaton A.** Respiratory and allergic symptoms in wool textile workers. *Br J Ind Med* 1988;45:727–741.

Source: *Occupational Medicine*, Volume 59, Issue 4, June 2009, Page 217, https://doi.org/10.1093/occmed/kqp064. Copyright © The Author 2009.
Reprinted by permission of Oxford University Press on behalf of the Society of Occupational Medicine.

Why I became an occupational physician ...

D. Coggon

Like many British occupational physicians, I discovered the specialty quite late in my career. Moreover, the route by which I got there hinged on a series of happy coincidences.

When I started my university education in Cambridge as a mathematician, I was interested in pursuing an academic career. It soon became clear that I did not have the ability to be a mathematical researcher, but a series of lectures on Markov methods, which included modelling the spread of infectious diseases, gave me the idea of trying to apply my mathematical skills in biological sciences. When I consulted my supervisor, he suggested that I switch to medicine. Not having done any biology since 'O levels' I had not appreciated that this was an option, but it seemed like a good idea, and having checked that the anatomy dissecting room was tolerable, I took the chance. My transfer to Oxford for my clinical undergraduate training exposed me to the epidemiologists there, in particular Martin Vessey with whom I spent my elective. From that time I was set on a career in epidemiology.

My first house job was in Southampton where I had the good fortune to work with two more epidemiologists, Donald Acheson and David Barker, both also physicians. Their advice was that I should undertake clinical training in internal medicine and get the MRCP before moving on to epidemiological research. Fortune again favoured me when I worked as a registrar for Michael Langman, another clinician with a strong interest in epidemiology, at the City Hospital in Nottingham. It was Michael who drew my attention to a post advertised in the newly established MRC Environmental Epidemiology Unit in Southampton. My intention had been to undertake a PhD in Nottingham in gastroenterology, but the opportunity was too good to miss, and I returned to Southampton to work under the guidance of Donald Acheson. For 3 months, I explored the possibility of working on an epidemiological study of breast cancer in young women or of melanoma, but finally we agreed that occupational risks of cancer would be the best bet.

At this stage, I was still unaware of occupational medicine as a clinical specialty, but my eyes were opened a couple of years later when I was asked to contribute to a presentation at an SOM meeting in London. From then I never looked back. Given my developing research interests and my clinical background in internal medicine, it was the natural choice for specialist training. With support and guidance from Oscar Lavanchy, Ivan Johnson and David Leitch, I arranged attachments with British Gas and HSE and completed the MFOM.

It is a choice that I have never regretted, but I am conscious of the luck that took me there. The irony is that had I been a better mathematician, I might have ended up doing similar research but without the added stimulus and variety of clinical work, and for a significantly lower salary.

Source: *Occupational Medicine*, Volume 55, Issue 8, December 2005, Page 585, https://doi.org/10.1093/occmed/kqi167. Copyright © The Author 2005.

Reprinted by permission of Oxford University Press on behalf of the Society of Occupational Medicine.

Coming to the end of the road in occupational health—lessons from cancer care

Naomi Brecker and Barbara Wren

Our hospital regularly organizes 'Schwartz rounds', open to all clinical staff as a forum to reflect on the emotional impact of difficult or troubling patients. The environment is safe and structured and the empathetic support of fellow health care workers is a powerful tool for group learning.

At yesterday's round, I listened to a joint presentation by an oncologist, a counsellor and a psychiatrist who each described their frustration and feelings of failure over a mutual patient. This was a young woman with metastatic disease who despite new treatments that offered prolonged life expectancy with a reduction in side effects plus psychological intervention was perceived as pessimistic in her world view. To the health professionals, it felt as if she made no attempt to gain control over her remaining few years of life. I was struck with the similarities with 'no hope' consultations in occupational health. You may recognize those clients who are failing in their jobs and for whom life outside work is difficult; they do not get on well with their managers who they accuse of bullying for managing poor performance; they do not get on with their colleagues; there are poor team dynamics as a result of their underperformance. This situation is inevitably stressful for all and limited resilience underpins the overt display of psychological distress in your client, who may already (or soon will be) signed off sick by their GP with 'workplace stress'. They have done nothing to help themselves out of a progressively difficult situation at work and look to occupational health to solve their problems.

So what are the similarities with the patient dying of cancer and what lessons can we learn from cancer care? The client in occupational health undoubtedly has a poor prognosis in their current role in the absence of any interventions. However with limitations to what occupational health can do, the possible options all have potential 'side effects'. We can support choices, but inevitably trade-offs will have to be made, just like in cancer care. As in cancer care using psychological frameworks to inform occupational health practice has the potential to benefit our difficult consultations. Despite this, some people will still choose to succumb to the inevitable. For these clients, if we have done our best and offered all the help that constrained resources will allow, we need to be able to let go. For the young woman with cancer, her glass remained half empty for two years before the disease took its inevitable course. Her clinicians acted as sounding boards for her negativity and anger but felt they had failed to improve her lot. In occupational health, we also have to face up to unhappy outcomes, but helping people to let go can be a positive result. Psychological frameworks can help us to manage consultations when options seem very limited, and to choose how best to intervene when patients seem unable to change. Sometimes we also need help in letting go!

Source: *Occupational Medicine*, Volume 61, Issue 1, January 2011, Page 61, https://doi.org/10.1093/occmed/kqq180. Copyright © The Author 2010.

Fifty years ago: 'The medical officer of health and the small workplace'

A.W.W. Robinson

Given at the Annual Provincial Meeting on 15 July 1964.

Up to the present time, the promotion and care of the health of the man or woman at work has been mostly confined to the large industrial organizations, the bigger of the commercial units such as banks and insurance companies, and a small handful of pioneer group health services. Even this favoured minority of workers is not given a uniform standard of occupational health cover, for apart from certain dangerous occupations, the standard depends very much on the enlightenment of the employer and whether the doctor really understands what is implied by the term 'occupational medicine'.

At last year's Provincial Meeting, we were given by Dr Bob Murray a most lucid and informative description of occupational health services in other countries of Europe. This opened my eyes (as it must have opened the eyes of many of us) to the extent by which we in this country have fallen behind. Whatever your views may be about Great Britain's entry to the Common Market, you must admit that we are not going to get away with ad hoc occupational health coverage for very much longer. Our patchy set-up is unlikely to be accepted by future partners in the European Economic Community as even an approximation to the International Labour Organization's Recommendation No. 112 on which the occupational health policy of the Six is based.

Assuming then that occupational health cover is to be given to every worker in the land, how is this to be done? Occupational medicine was left out of the original National Health Service plan because domestic and curative medicine were given priority and because there was no model on which a national occupational health service could be based. This has meant that the National Health Service crystallized into its present form without an occupational health component.

I think that there is little doubt that the politically convenient policy of allowing a national occupational health service to be evolved by voluntary extension has failed, as it was bound to do. But before we discuss any alternative to the purely laissez faire policy, I should like to try to establish what the functions and shape of an occupational health service are—at least what I think they are, for opinions are by no means unanimous about this. I see the function of such a service as being the promotion of the health of the worker, in its widest sense, during working hours. I see occupational medicine as complementary to preventive and curative medicine, performing some of the functions of the former, appreciably fewer of the functions of the latter, but with also its own special part to play in the life of the individual worker. It is a mistake to think of Medicine as being divided into compartments.

Source: *Occupational Medicine*, Volume 64, Issue 5, July 2014, Page 386, https://doi.org/10.1093/occmed/kqu031. Copyright © The Author 2014.

Originally from: The medical officer of health and the small workplace. *Trans Ass Industr Med Offrs* (1964) 14, 75. Available at: *Occupational Medicine*, Volume 14, Issue 1, 1 April 1964, Pages 75–78.

The human spirit level

John Hobson

'It's not level' she announced having tottered in and sat down, husband in tow. Elegant, immaculately presented, attractive. I knew that the next half hour would be occupied by a detailed description of her every symptom and difficulty as she made her case for her pension, her hang-dog husband interjecting the occasional supporting statement but for the most part looking as if he was thoroughly fed up. My heart sank a little at the prospect of the next 30 minutes.

'Your floor. It's not level.' She proceeded to tell me about the undulations in the floor between the waiting area and the consultation room that I had never noticed and how the 5-metre journey had left her reeling and nauseous. She looked surprisingly well and not green despite the tricky terrain she had negotiated to come and see me. When out shopping she had to cling onto walls and street furniture; her embarrassed children would shout at her, 'Mum, stop it!' Her animated description of the uneven surface of her world prompted a smile if only internally on that side of my face the patient never sees, the one facing my mind, her lively depiction of her rolling world an unexpected bonus from a chore consultation. A visit inside a pink and stationary caravan had left her unwell for days, bed ridden and unable to drive her car, her shopping trips and visits to the library impossible.

'I'm like a spirit level; a human spirit level.'

The label stuck in my mind. Here was a woman who described herself as a rectangular piece of wood, straight and regular, rigid but for the ever restless bubble relentlessly seeking higher ground and a more comfortable place. Her neatness and sense of order was constantly challenged as her bubble budged this way then that with every successive step, always on a playing field that never was. Slopes were steep inclines, ripples were waves, molehills were mountains. The contour chaos of her world had not only disrupted her sense of level but her sense of perspective. The balance of her life had tipped.

We are all spirit levels. We have our own sense of what is smooth and even, where we want to be and when things are out. Our bubbles normally behave; hers had burst and scattered like a lava lamp, Brownian and bouncy, randomly seeking out different planes. A physical correction was beyond medical science but more importantly she needed something to help level her spirit, to return a sense of order to her life, to rebalance her perspective rather than her perpendicular. I hope she finds out how but I doubt it. As the consultation ended on its usual unsatisfactory note I once again suggested the potential benefits of therapy; her husband resignedly nodded in silent agreement. As I followed them out of the room and she tottered away into the corridor, I tilted my head and gazed along the floor to see if I had missed anything.

Source: *Occupational Medicine*, Volume 62, Issue 8, December 2012, Page 599, https://doi.org/10.1093/occmed/kqs086. Copyright © The Author 2012.

Why I became an occupational physician …

R. Ian McCallum

Pulmonary tuberculosis, as a student, turned me to lung diseases as a specialty, so after house jobs at Guy's Hospital and the Brompton Hospital, and some locum work in the tuberculosis service which was then in decline, I went to Newcastle upon Tyne to a new department of Industrial Health to study pneumoconiosis of coal workers. The Department, which was funded by the Nuffield Foundation and welcomed by local physicians, was innovative. Under the late Richard Browne teaching of undergraduates occupational health, medical statistics, pulmonary physiology; social workers instead of the older lady almoners, and record keeping were introduced so that it has become a major school of medicine.

My post involved research and teaching in occupational medicine to undergraduate medical students, and over the next 25 years, I worked on pneumoconiosis (in conjunction with the Unit at Cardiff), lead poisoning, antimony toxicology, compressed air disease (when the Tyne Tunnels were built) and eventually the long-term effects of diving (especially bone necrosis). Although to my regret, I never took a DIH, I was so involved in the area that I was awarded an MRC Rockefeller Fellowship which took me to Pittsburgh, USA, and was editor of the *British Journal of Industrial Medicine* for 7 years; president of the SOM, the BOHS and the Section of Occupational Medicine of the RSM; Dean of the Faculty of Occupational Medicine 1984–6; Professor of Occupational Medicine and Hygiene at Newcastle University and civilian adviser to the army from 1980–6 among other tasks. Thus, I came into the specialty by default and out of interest in what I was doing.

At the time occupational disease was not uncommon and the field was a largely clinical one so that an MRCP was an advantage. I sense that the field has changed a good deal during the last few years and occupational disease may not be so important as it was. Since retirement, I have become involved in medical historical studies, particularly in the Scottish alchemists of the 17th century, but I still gave a paper in Heidelberg on antimony toxicity last year.

Source: *Occupational Medicine*, Volume 57, Issue 3, May 2007, Page 226, https://doi.org/10.1093/occmed/kql079. Copyright © The Author 2007.

A close friend

David Walker

A close friend of mine has had a varied medical life. Laboratory researcher, university lecturer, epidemiologist and for the second half of his time in the National Health Service, a clinician trying to manage illness and rehabilitation in older people. Many older people, he tells me, are fit, while others simply flirt with frailty. Stands to reason if they have survived thus far. Importantly, he saw it as a window on his own future. Around the age of 50, life and work events overwhelmed him and a career break seemed a sensible way forward. He returned to university and, for the next two years, studied behavioural sciences, completing a master's dissertation on the forces that encourage and inhibit midlife change. Unsurprisingly, he discovered that change tends to be sudden, brought on by events that are difficult to control, such as illness and redundancy, and the main impact is on the job.

Very few plan for change apparently. I have often wondered about doctors' needs for transformation with age. We are not as physically capable in our 50s and 60s. Skills based on strength, stamina and eyesight for instance cannot go on forever. Long operating lists and demanding emergency duties are no longer a welcome challenge. Yet the experience and intellect are still there. Transformation, cashing in on lifelong intellectual property and networks, needs advance thought, before people get too tired to bother and simply settle for seeing out their time to the pension. My friend catalogued some of the forces acting on this process. A passionate interest, a personal skill, constraining rules, tiring paperwork and adapting to incessant change would be examples of influences that might push people into a move. On the other hand, yet more rules bound up in the fear of relative poverty pull them back into staying as they are.

My friend describes careers as the spokes of a wheel. It is much easier to transform to a closely related activity, an adjacent spoke, rather than jump across to an unfamiliar part of the wheel. Doctors adapt successfully to part-time work in outpatients, they make good teachers and some enter management, but very few become airline pilots. The government wants men and women on incapacity benefit back in work. What of those who are still clocking in but not actually working? What about a strategy for transformation instead of planning for retirement? My friend concedes it may not apply to everyone. Manual workers can struggle. Crippling illness can be a major barrier. And there are those with underdeveloped personal resources where the problem and solution sit firmly in someone else's lap. These are challenging, but not insurmountable. He also concedes if people have enough income to get by, they may transform out of the workforce altogether, doing voluntary work, writing, painting or whatever they are passionate about. It is still work after all. What did my friend do? He became an occupational health physician.

Source: *Occupational Medicine*, Volume 58, Issue 8, December 2008, Page 583, https://doi.org/10.1093/occmed/kqn102. Copyright © The Author 2008.

Occupational hazard of rubber tapping

J.T. Mets

An occupational hazard to rubber tappers in the forests of Sumatra, Indonesia, is the risk of being attacked by a tiger. Collecting rubber is done by making a small cut in the bark of a tree, then fixing a small metal 'gutter and cup' right under the cut. Latex trickling down into the cups is collected later and dried in the sun to form large rubber 'slabs'. While at work one morning, two young men were attacked by a tiger when 'tapping' rubber in a forest far away from the hospital I was in charge of at the time (1959).

On arrival, one casualty was semi-comatose. The tiger had hit him on the right side of his head; this had caused a temporal bone fracture, displaced inwards, with torn skin pulled down over the ear. Liquor and blood were oozing from the wound.

His colleague told us how it had happened: his friend had squatted next to a tree to relieve himself when a tiger, coming from behind this, had struck him. He himself had jumped to his friend's aid and had hit the tiger with his heavy golok (chopper). The tiger had then turned on him pawing his right shoulder, pulling down skin and muscle, inflicting a gaping wound. His loud screaming and shouting had caused the tiger to flee when other rubber tappers nearby came to their aid. Hidden in this simple account is the courage of this young rubber tapper to attack a tiger, thereby saving his friend's life! It took the men two days to reach our hospital, transporting two casualties first by boat, then carrying them along the road.

Surgical intervention to the first man consisted of cleaning the wound under local anaesthesia, lifting the temporal bone fragment up to re-align it, suturing the galea aponeurotica, excising suspected non-viable tissue and closing the wound, with a soft drain in place. Anti-tetanus serum was administered and aureomycin intravenously for some days. Once in the ward, the man soon regained full consciousness.

The other young man I treated by cleaning the wound, instilling antibiotic fluid, suturing muscle, fascia and skin, administering anti-tetanus serum and then antibiotics for a few days. Nursing care made him recover within a week, able to go home. His more seriously injured mate took much longer.

When eventually friends came to collect him to return home, he walked away from us with a bright smile on his face and much waving of the hand, saying 'Terima kasih banyak' ('I thank you very much') a dozen times! No doubt both men will much later have enjoyed telling a tall tale to family and friends!

Acknowledgements

I acknowledge Shell International Medical Services, who enabled me to treat this occupational injury by providing me with a well-equipped and staffed hospital, boasting the only operative Surgical Theatre in an area with a radius of 200 km.

Tales of Kieran: The occupational physician's odyssey 3—The Birdman of Linbridge

J.A. Hunter

It's absolutely ages since I last saw Kieran so when I happened to be at Linbridge University the other week I called into the Occupational Health Department. I opened his office door to be blinded by a very bright light. As my pupils adjusted I found myself staring down the barrel of a gun. The light suddenly went out, my retinas recovered and Kieran appeared at the other end.

'What on earth ... '

'Bird shit' said Kieran calmly, oblivious to the fact that my myocardium was still contemplating fibrillation. 'Droppings, guano ... ' he continued as I came to the conclusion that making a run for it was obviously the best option as Kieran had finally gone really mad. 'Psittacosis' he said finally which for some reason seemed to make everything alright. I returned to the sinus rhythm although still not sure what was happening.

'We've had an outbreak of psittacosis' explained Kieran 'well, a case at least. One of the University maintenance engineers has had quite a nasty illness two weeks after clearing up pigeon droppings in one of the boiler houses. We did a COSHH assessment on the stuff and managed to grow *Clamydia*. A survey of the other maintenance men has shown a lot of unexplained upper respiratory tract symptoms. So in accordance with EC Directive 91/784 we are going to try and eradicate the problem.'

'What, kill the pigeons?' I exclaimed as my attention was caught by the cardboard cutout hawk in the window.

'Yes of course. You can use the fun with the light at night whilst they are all still sleeping. But listen to this!'

Kieran fiddled with a black box on his desk and I leapt out of my skin as the room was suddenly filled by high-pitched shrieking noises.

'Impressive isn't it? That's a PAL Sound Emitter; makes the pigeons think there's a hawk about, like the cardboard cutouts. Soon have the blighters eradicated' Kieran shouted gleefully waving the gun around as if he had just shot a lion. My shattered nervous system could stand no more so I made the excuses and left Kieran to his plans for mass avicide.

A couple of weeks later I found myself at the University again and was pleased to note encouraging signs of persistent birdlife. More importantly the peace of the campus was not punctuated by the sounds of the searchlight-guided elephant gun or the high-pitched shrieking of recorded birds of prey. Nonetheless I decided to check with Jeanne first before entering Kieran's office in case he was trying out a ground-to-air missile of some other weapon of pigeon destruction.

Jeanne solemnly advised against it. 'He's as sick as a parrot' she said with a very straight face. 'A very sad example of mouth-to-break resuscitation.'

'Mouth-to-beak resuscitation?' I said incredulously.

'Kieran's "case" of psittacosis got wind of this plans to rid the University of all bird life. So he admitted to Kieran that he was an exotic bird importer in his spare time. His last bird arrived in this country moribund and the birds are so expensive that he tried to resuscitate it.'

As I left I noticed workmen in Kieran's office replacing a pane of glass and on the floor what looked suspiciously like the cardboard cut-out of a hawk that had been shot several times. As I'm always telling the medical students, never underestimate the importance of taking a proper history!

Source: *Occupational Medicine,* Volume 52, Issue 4, June 2002, Page 231, https://doi.org/10.1093/occmed/52.4.231. Copyright © Society of Occupational Medicine 2002.

Reprinted with permission from Hunter J. A. (1993). *Lancet.* 342(886):301.

Hunting canaries

Mike Gibson

As one of the surgical consultants at medical school warned, 'Sparrows are commoner than canaries'. But the case I have in mind followed a series of canaries, so I was in full canary-spotting mode. The differential diagnosis of red eye does not usually include being stabbed in the eye by an unpeeled banana. Then there was the airman who was attacked by a screaming rabbit while he was cycling home from work. And the little girl who had to be freed when the cinema seat she had been sitting on flipped. At the time, one of my hospital roles was to head the Board deciding medical categories for RAF personnel in Germany. The particular patient that day had noticed a lump under his left arm 4 years before. Biopsy proved it to be an anaplastic secondary melanoma. He had a block dissection of the axilla. Intensive investigation, including whole body screening, failed to discover any primary. A year later, he had a lump under the other arm. Biopsy this time showed reactive hyperplasia.

Now, a further 3 years later and still well, he wanted to be able to return to his specialist role as a parachute jumping instructor. On taking his history, I noticed that his glasses were extremely clean, unlike my usually dusty and smeared lenses. He confirmed that they were new but said that they were not very good, particularly the right eye. On looking with the ophthalmoscope I could only see grey fuzz. I dropped the blinds and turned out the lights. Still only grey fuzz. The canaries started chirping. I knew about melanoma of the choroid, but could you have amelanotic melanoma of the choroid? Fortunately, we had a consultant ophthalmologist just down the corridor and, intrigued by the story, he saw him immediately. Within 5 minutes, I had my answer. The patient had a mature cataract. Which only goes to show that, as a late Texan colleague of mine put it: 'The hoofbeats you hear outside your window are usually horses, not zebras'.

Source: *Occupational Medicine*, Volume 64, Issue 8, December 2014, Page 634, https://doi.org/10.1093/occmed/kqu086. Copyright © The Author 2014.

Reprinted by permission of Oxford University Press on behalf of the Society of Occupational Medicine.

Why I became an occupational physician …

William Dixon

It was the discovery by Selman Waksman of streptomycin in 1944 that eventually led me to a drastic change of career at the relatively late age of 35 years. As a medical student at Guy's, I had contracted pulmonary tuberculosis and was still, in 1949, 2 years after qualifying, unable to work a full day. Like many other doctors, the only career open to me was life in a sanatorium. I was fortunate in landing a job at Tor-na-Dee, working under the charismatic Bobby (RY) Keers. When I had recovered sufficiently to work full time, he pushed me out to Birmingham Chest Clinic, the RCP Membership and a job as a Senior Registrar in London and eventually an SHMO job at the Hammersmith where I came under the spell of the great Charles Fletcher. Consultant jobs in chest medicine soon dried up as BCG and the newer antibiotics, like streptomycin, brought tuberculosis under control. In the 1920s, many Welsh miners had migrated to West London and brought with them their miners' pneumoconiosis and pulmonary tuberculosis. I had visited the Pneumoconiosis Research Unit at Cardiff and was fascinated—so thought I would make a career in industrial lung disease research.

When I saw an advertisement for an occupational physician at ESSO, Fawley, I applied thinking (i) that I would walk it and (ii) that I would do it for a couple of years before returning to a job in respiratory research. Neither prediction was correct! But I did get the job and never regretted the move. The most surprising element was that I was dealing with colleagues who were quite well and neither patients nor other doctors. My opinions were questioned by highly qualified chemists, engineers, personnel managers and tough-talking American construction men who stood no nonsense. When I was given my own department to run at ESSO, Milford Haven, all thoughts of a return to the National Health Service (NHS) disappeared. I had my first major emergency when the first super-tanker caught fire at the berth, but our preparations stood the test; I learnt the importance of teamwork and delegation. When the construction crews left, we had too few people to justify my staying on so I moved to Scotland, then to Fisons and after a short period as CMO of Chrysler, UK, I was made redundant. I often remind colleagues in the NHS that we may get paid more but we take bigger career risks! I spent the last years of my professional life as Head of Medical Services for the John Lewis Partnership, including Waitrose. To my pleasant surprise, the health problems in the retail and food industry were just as protean as in any other industry. In retrospect, it was the sheer variety of tasks in occupational medicine which constantly retained my enthusiasm—no two days the same and like many others in a small speciality I enjoyed the fruits of office in various professional societies—not least the dear old SOM. So no regrets and many blessings.

Source: *Occupational Medicine*, Volume 57, Issue 3, May 2007, Page 231, https://doi.org/10.1093/occmed/kql080. Copyright © The Author 2007.

Why I now watch my step as an occupational physician …

James Preston

As an occupational physician, like many readers, I see people with temporary or permanent impairments. We can use the biopsychosocial model to assess presentation, but how truly do we understand the impact of impairment on an individual's life?

I have the opportunity to reflect on an experience, recall the impact and seek to learn from it.

I live in a split-level London flat. I was a keen badminton player until one evening I tore my medial ankle ligament (grade 2) and lateral ligament (grade 1).

I could not weight-bear through that foot for 2 weeks and was partially weight-bearing for a further 6 weeks.

From being a busy, outgoing person things changed overnight. Living alone, every aspect of life was affected. I would bottom shuffle around my flat. I could not carry a cup from kitchen to living room. I could not stand in the shower. A journey to the local shop took 40 minutes instead of 5 minutes. 'Simple' tasks were suddenly overwhelming.

Crucially, this impairment had a profound effect on my relationship with the outside world. I was moving in slow motion. I could not identify with those who were rushing, carefree, distracted.

I had no choice but to take time; using crutches, using lifts in tube stations (try using crutches on an escalator, time the hop-off at the end and then move on before people behind pile on top of you). I had a near panic attack in rush hour tube conditions.

I was unprepared for the response of strangers. I was offered seats on trains and buses; but I felt guilty. Once, I asked for a seat on the tube because no-one offered. The man relented but with a look of contempt. There was no consistency with how people responded which was very disarming.

I started judging friends on how much effort they made to keep in touch; often my socializing is done by meeting 'centrally' and not home visiting. I had far less human contact. I could not manage central London meeting places. This triggered negative thinking patterns about life in London and my sense of 'community' and identity.

I felt so lucky to have a temporary impairment and my crises have passed. I did not miss a day at work thanks to the kindness and flexibility of colleagues and customers alike.

I learnt how profound the impact can be of something that makes one 'different' from the ordinary person. I learnt that a host of minor inconveniences lead to a major effect on 'capacity'. What one can do in theory becomes unrealistic in practice. The additional effort to manage is exhausting and mentally draining.

As occupational health practitioners, we need to understand the human experience of people when we have to judge fitness; particularly in the context of determining permanent incapacity for pension purposes. I am not sure my experience makes that easier, so much as highlights how complex it is to make a robust assessment.

Source: *Occupational Medicine*, Volume 62, Issue 1, January 2012, Page 40, https://doi.org/10.1093/occmed/kqr155. Copyright © The Author 2011.

Reprinted by permission of Oxford University Press on behalf of the Society of Occupational Medicine.

Fifty years ago: 'Occupational health: An employer's view'

R. Viner

Given at the Annual Provincial Meeting on 15 July 1964.

To me as a layman and an employing manufacturer, occupational health in a factory conjures up immediately the idea of accidents, hazard prevention and dealing with emergencies. I feel it is most important that industrial medical officers should appreciate the layman's point of view. Evidently, however, this symposium covers not only these aspects but the promotion and maintenance of good health generally amongst those occupied for so great a part of their lives in a workplace, and in the context of these discussions, a small workplace. Hence it naturally follows that our deliberations must cover a very wide field, including prompt and adequate treatment of all accidents, hazard prevention, cleanliness and hygiene, as well as pleasant surroundings, and, of particular importance, the education of both workpeople and employers in the principles of health maintenance.

It is singularly opportune that such a conference should be held in Sheffield, where there are many small workplaces, as in most areas of long-established industrialization. Although vast improvements have taken place in recent years, many of these are quite inadequate from a health point of view.

This is not the occasion to sit back and bask in the sunshine of our achievements; this symposium provides a platform to emphasize these inadequacies and gives the opportunity for suggestions for rectification. As an example, I would like to give some particulars of my own industry, which I am afraid is quite typical. Not so very long ago this comprised some 600 units employing about 12 000 people; the 1959 statistics give 450 units employing some 11 000, of which there were 186 firms with one to five workers. I am pleased to say that we are now down to some 300, but obviously there is still much scope for improvement. I understand that over 22% of the manufacturing establishments in the country employ between 11 and 24 people, and a further 50% between 25 and 100.

Many of these small places simply cannot make the necessary provision of healthy working conditions. I do not feel that it is right we should accept the plea of poverty as an excuse—if a firm cannot provide adequate facilities for its workpeople, it should not be in business, nor should the suitability, age or dilapidation of premises be an excuse for unsatisfactory conditions. Such places should not be licensed as suitable for people to work in.

With the establishment of factory estates and the zoning of industry, I think it would be a helpful and paying proposition for centres to be established at a distance of not more than about 5 or 10 min away from any one workplace. These should be staffed with a nurse and person qualified to deal with first aid, the necessary equipment to cover its requirements, a rest room and, if possible, an ambulance. If the cost of these centres was put on a per capita basis for the firms using them, I do not think it would be too high for any individual concern, and in any case by preventing, as I am sure it would, the loss of many working hours, be a paying proposition.

Source: *Occupational Medicine,* Volume 64, Issue 6, September 2014, Page 467, https://doi.org/10.1093/occmed/kqu032. Copyright © The Author 2014.

Originally from: Occupational health: An employer's view. *Trans Ass Industr Med Offrs* (1964) 14, 79. Available at: *Occup Med (Lond)* 1964;14:79–80. DOI:10.1093/ occmed/14.1.79.

Clinical research

Anthony Seaton

'What sort of scientist are you?' asked my colleague, a physicist. 'Well, I suppose I'm a clinical scientist.' And then I started to wonder what that meant. It was not too complicated in the old days. If, like most readers of this journal, you were a clinician, your patients threw up questions to which you did not know the answer. You spent a bit of time in the library going through Index Medicus and read the relevant articles. You would be lucky if you got what you wanted on the first visit, as those old journals would throw up such interesting, forgotten papers on other subjects that you spent a lot of time reading them instead. This would now be called CPE, but then we just thought of it as SNC, satisfaction of natural curiosity. But sometimes you realized that you did not know the answer because nobody else did, so you set out trying to find out. In my field, the interesting opportunities at that time were in physiology, so we collected our patients, asked them nicely if they would be prepared to help and measured whatever it was. We asked our colleagues and friends if they would mind acting as controls. The introduction of ethics committees after the very necessary strictures by Maurice Papworth in 'Human Guinea Pigs' did not hinder this sort of activity but imposed a desirable discipline on the process. Some of my friends preferred immunology, others genetics, but in essence, we all did the same sort of thing, alongside our heavy clinical responsibilities and without any thought as to the hours we worked.

Most of us did not realize that in doing this, we had moved in a completely different direction to that in which we were trained. The practice of medicine requires the accumulation of a large amount of knowledge, the general understanding of the workings of the human body, which we then apply to the specific problems raised by the individual patient, a process of deductive logic. In becoming a researcher, we turn this process on its head, investigating the particular issues raised by our patients in order to draw general conclusions that might be applied in their future management and treatment, an inductive process. So the trained scientist understandably may be confused by the term 'clinical scientist'. Few of us had any formal scientific training; we picked it up.

Clinical science has now changed. Often it requires large laboratories, complicated equipment and teams of research fellows. It tends to be dominated by non-medically qualified scientists, some of whom have little understanding of public health or even pathology. But at its heart, if it is to contribute to improvement of the health of people, must be the clinical question, the question arising at the bedside about our patients. The word clinical, after all, means related to the bed.

Source: *Occupational Medicine*, Volume 59, Issue 7, October 2009, Page 505, https://doi.org/10.1093/occmed/kqp065. Copyright © The Author 2009.

Why I became an occupational physician …

David Snashall

As a schoolboy, I often worked during my holidays—painting and decorating (I once painted part of Buckingham Palace), forest work in Wales, as a wool sorter and in a timber yard where I fell off a stack and broke my wrist. My worst job was in an insurance office. I went down a coal mine in Yorkshire which was terrifying and as a medical student in Edinburgh visited a factory making tractor tyres by hand which was even worse.

After house jobs in Warwick, Paris and Edinburgh where Professor John Gillingham told me politely I would never be a neurosurgeon, I did MRCP and moved to Canada where I worked as a doctor in logging camps, asbestos and tungsten mines.

I had set my mind on going to South America so learned Spanish and wrote to President Allende of Chile asking him to give me a job, which he did but his untimely demise days before I was due to cross the border from Bolivia brought that plan to an end.

I came back to Britain, worked briefly in general practice then replied to an advertisement for a Spanish-speaking British doctor to set up medical services for the Majes project in Peru. This, one of the largest hydro-irrigation schemes in the world, was dramatic and the infrastructure was poor. We travelled on mule for the first few months, some of the work was >4000 m in altitude and I was one of the only two expatriate doctors.

Accidents were terrible due to bad roads, weather and reckless driving and conditions on the dams and in the hard rock tunnels were appalling. Occupational lung and skin disorders and public health problems of dysentery, scabies and sexually transmitted diseases were rife in the 4000 strong local workforce. The expatriates suffered culture shock, high altitude disorders and drank too much. I was given much support in my amateurish efforts to cope with all this by Griffith Pugh, the physiologist who designed the oxygen supply for the 1953 Everest Expedition.

Encouraged by him, I came back to Britain in 1977 with an interest in environmental physiology but then came under the influence of Richard Schilling, Corbett McDonald and Bob Murray at the London School of Hygiene. This was my introduction to occupational medicine and how to do it properly.

I did the MSc/DIH course and the diploma in tropical medicine and spent a year working in Africa trying to apply what I had learned. St Thomas' was a logical next step!

I have never really planned my career, just tried to make the best of chances as they came up. I once read that Alexander Fleming had the same approach: looking back on those moments in his life when he could have gone in one direction or another, he invariably made the choice for reasons which, later, seemed trivial. I have the same philosophy. I did not discover penicillin but have been lucky enough to have an exciting, varied and fulfilling medical career.

Source: *Occupational Medicine*, Volume 57, Issue 4, June 2007, Page 237, https://doi.org/10.1093/occmed/kql112. Copyright © The Author 2007.

Reprinted by permission of Oxford University Press on behalf of the Society of Occupational Medicine.

The RMS Titanic

Ken Addley and Paul McKeagney

April 10th 2012 marks the centenary of the maiden voyage of the Royal Mail Ship Titanic—the most famous ship to have been built by the Harland and Wolff Shipyard in Belfast and commemorated with an iconic exhibition centre on the site of the original building dock.

When Harland and Wolff (H & W) was founded in 1858, Belfast was emerging as a major industrial centre with shipbuilding complementing factory-based linen production and at its peak, employed up to 20 000 workers [1,2]. The White Star Line commissioned the Titanic, one of the three luxury ocean liners known as 'Olympic-class'. Titanic was steel-hulled, 882.5 feet long, 42 238 tonnes, had 46 000 horsepower, a speed of 21 knots, a capacity to carry 3547 passengers and crew and cost £1.5 million [3,4]. Construction started in March 1909 and the ship was completed 3 years and 3 million steel rivets later.

Titanic left Belfast on 2nd April 1912 and after taking on passengers and crew, it departed Southampton on 10th April 1912 on its maiden voyage bound for New York (Figure 56.1). There were two stops en route to embark and disembark passengers, at Cherbourg in France and Queenstown (now Cobh) in Cork, before heading out into the Atlantic Ocean. The liner was two thirds of full capacity with 2206 people on board. On the night of the 14th April, the ship struck an iceberg at 11.40 pm sustaining a 300-foot gash to the hull, sinking within 3 hours at 2.20 a.m. on 15th April with the loss of 1514 lives—mostly male passengers and crew members [5]. Titanic, with 16 lifeboats, exceeded the outdated regulatory quota for British ships at the time. The boats could accommodate 1178 people—enough for just over half of those on board. Even with that limited capacity, the boats were not full and there were 705 survivors [5].

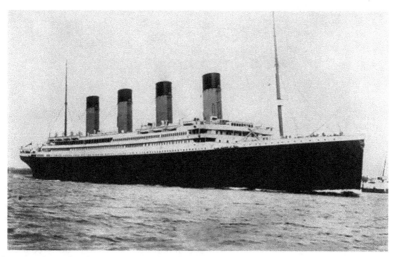

Figure 56.1 Titanic at Southampton, 7 April 1912

Reproduced with permission. Copyright © National Museums Northern Ireland Collection Ulster Folk and Transport Museum.

The British Board of Inquiry blamed the captain for failing to heed ice warnings. The Board of Trade was censured for inadequate lifeboat and watertight hull subdivision regulations. Other recommendations included: manning of lifeboats; lifeboat drills; top to bottom watertight bulkheads and double skin hulls. H & W was praised for its workmanship and exonerated of any culpability [6].

Shipyard work was heavy and hazardous and in the early 1900s, health and safety had a low priority. There were many physical hazards: falls from heights, injury from falling objects and crushing by machinery and/or materials—eight deaths occurred in the building of the Titanic mostly due to falls [5]. Exposure to heavy manual work, awkward postures and long working hours were associated with a range of musculoskeletal conditions [7]. Noise-induced deafness/tinnitus and vibration white finger were common (Figure 56.2) [8].

Welding fume, nitrous oxide, solvents, lead, mercurials and isocyanates were potentially carcinogenic, teratogenic and asthma inducing. Anoxia, asphyxiation and explosion were associated with confined spaces [8].

More than 1000 tons of asbestos was used as boiler insulation annually between 1906 and 1923 [9]. The hazardous nature of asbestos was not recognized until the 1930s following reports of lung fibrosis in those heavily exposed, often coexisting with tuberculosis infection and smoking-related symptoms [10]. Little protection was deployed and exposure extended to families from contaminated clothing. It took many years, and many shipyard workers' deaths, for the link between asbestos exposure and pleural mesothelioma to become apparent [11–14]. In 1955, Doll described increased mortality from lung cancer in asbestos workers and the additive effect of smoking [15]. The rate of asbestos bodies present in the Belfast population in the 1960s was up

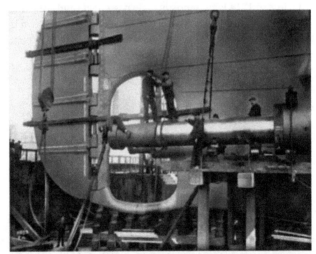

Figure 56.2 Titanic—fitting starboard tail propeller shaft prior to launch, 1911. The Titanic was powered by two large reciprocating steam engines and a central steam turbine. The cast-steel rudder, constructed in six sections, had two independent engines and was moved by telemotors from the bridge or by mechanical means from the docking bridge. There were three propellers (built in England by the Darlington Forge Company)—two wing shafts were 0.7 m in diameter and the central shaft 0.5 m. The propellers themselves, made of manganese bronze, had three blades each—on the wing 7 m in diameter and centrally 5 m.

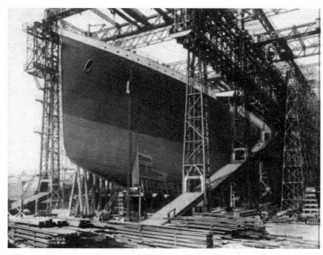

Figure 56.3 Titanic—port bow view on slipway in preparation for launch into Belfast Lough on 31 May 1911. After being launched, it took a year of fitting out and sea trials before Titanic left Belfast for Southampton. The hull was constructed of large steel plating sheets measuring 17 m² each with the overlapping panels triple riveted. Hydraulic riveting equipment, a new technology at the time, was used for some of this work. During the construction, there were eight deaths, 28 workers sustained severe injuries and there were 218 other injuries. Fatalities were mostly due to falls followed by crush injury. Of the deaths, six occurred on or around the ship during construction and fitting out and two in the workshops and sheds.

to 20% [16], suggesting a large proportion were exposed to significant environmental levels of asbestos [17].

The Titanic story provides a valuable lesson highlighting the need to anticipate, recognize, eliminate and control hazards; to have safe systems of work and adequate training; the potential that materials being used may have long latency health risk and avoidance of complacency and learning from mistakes to improve engineering design, working practices, safety and health. In conclusion, one hundred years on, the fact that the shortcomings of the Titanic era have been largely addressed is perhaps a fitting tribute to those workers, crew members and passengers who lost their lives due to their association with the vessel (Figure 56.3).

References

1. **Lynch JP.** An Unlikely Success Story: The Belfast Shipbuilding Industry 1880–1935. Belfast The Belfast Society, 2001.
2. **Johnston K.** In the Shadows of Giants: A Social History of the Belfast Shipyards. Dublin Gill & Macmillan, 2008.
3. **Moss MS, Hume JR.** Shipbuilders to the World: 125 years of Harland and Wolff, Belfast 1861–1986. Belfast Blackstaff Press, 1986.
4. **Dyos HJ, Aldcroft DW.** British Transport. Leicester: Leicester University Press, 1969; 244.
5. **Cameron S.** Titanic: Belfast's Own. Dublin Wolfhound Press, 1998.

6. British Wreck Commissioner's Inquiry, Report on the Loss of the "Titanic." London Board of Trade's Administration, 1912.

7. **Torell G, Sanden A.** Musculoskeletal disorders in shipyard workers. *Occup Med (Lond)* 1988;**38**:109–113.

8. **Wollaston JF.** Shipbuilding and ship repair. *Occup Med (Lond)* 1992;**42**:203–212.

9. **Elmes PC, McCaughey WTE, Wade OL.** Diffuse mesothelioma of the pleura and asbestos. *Br Med J* 1965;**1**:350–353.

10. **Cooke WE.** Pulmonary asbestosis. *Br Med J* 1927;**2**:1024–1027.

11. **Campbell SBB, Young JS.** A primary tumour (mixed cell sarcoma) of the pleura. *Ulster Med J* 1935;**4**:36–38.

12. **McCaughey WTE.** Primary tumours of the pleura. *J Pathol Bacteriol* 1928;**31**:265–275.

13. **Wagner J, Sleggs CA.** Diffuse pleural mesothelioma and asbestos exposure in the north western cape provence. *Br J Ind Med* 1960;**17**:260–271.

14. **Logan JS, Bharucha H, Sloan JM.** Mesotheliomas: long before their time. *Ulster Med J* 1996;**65**:1–2.

15. **Doll R.** Mortality from lung cancer in asbestos workers. *Br J Ind Med* 1955;**12**:81–86.

16. **Elmes PC.** Investigation into the hazardous use of asbestos: Northern Ireland 1960–1976. *Ulster Med J* 1977;**46**:71–80.

17. **Hedley-Whyte J, Milamed DR.** Asbestos and ship building: fatal consequences. *Ulster Med J* 2008;**77**:191–200.

Source: *Occupational Medicine*, Volume 62, Issue 3, April 2012, Pages 165–166, https://doi.org/10.1093/occmed/kqs015. © The Author 2012.

Reprinted by permission of Oxford University Press on behalf of the Society of Occupational Medicine.

Fifty years ago: 'Assessment of the ability to work of the "Unfit"'

Kenneth Lee

In the Apothecaries' Lecture given before this Society on 25 March last year, Doctor Lloyd Davies said: 'For every spell of sickness for which benefit is paid due to prescribed industrial diseases, there are three hundred spells from nonindustrial disease. The patient's general practitioner is responsible for determining fitness for work after an illness. No one would challenge this. Equally the majority of patients return to work successfully. There remains, however, a burden of distress where selected patients would be helped by skilled advice, not about their illness, but about how their work is affected by their illness. How big this burden is I do not know but I suspect it is very considerable.' I wish to discuss the question of return to work and responsibility for determining fitness for work after illness. At first glance it may be thought that there is no problem at all. As far as industry is concerned it is becoming more complex and the worker's tasks are becoming more selective and skilled. The worker is either able or unable to do his task. As far as the general practitioner is concerned the patient is either fit or unfit. This all seems quite straightforward and simple, so why should we challenge it? Do any of us believe that a man becomes fit overnight from a long and debilitating illness? At what stage during the patient's recovery should the general practitioner reach for his pen and sign the final certificate? What is fitness anyhow? A man may be unfit to be an airline pilot but this does not mean that he is unfit to do any work. Often it must be very difficult for the general practitioner to decide just when his patient may return to work and if he has little or no knowledge of the patient's work then the decision is an arbitrary one. In industry, it is much easier to have people coming back to work fully fit for their tasks. Everything is arranged for people to do certain tasks. Any adjustment or alteration of this is inconvenient and is often thought to be uneconomical. We reach a stage where a manager will say 'I don't want that man in through the factory gates until he is 100 per cent fit.' The social security system contributes to this problem. The worker is either fully fit for his full-time employment or is totally unfit and needs social security benefits. It seems that work is held to be a necessary evil and that we work only in order to eat. If we believe this is true then there is little wrong with the present system, but Garland reminded us in his paper on 'Fraser's Disease' that work provides many areas of satisfaction in our lives. I wish to base my argument on the premise that to want to work is normal. I want to show how one industry has evolved a system of providing a gradual return to work after illness, to show that this is a useful and perfectly practical measure and to argue that this is one of the most useful spheres of work for the industrial physician.

Source: *Occupational Medicine*, Volume 68, Issue 5, July 2018, Page 342, https://doi.org/10.1093/occmed/kqx196. Copyright © The Author(s) 2018.

Originally from: Assessment of the ability to work of the 'Unfit'. *Trans Soc Occup Med* (1968) 18, 61–65. Available at: *Occup Med (Lond)* 1968;18:61–66. DOI:10.1093/ occmed/18.1.61

In search of the black stuff

Kirstie Gibson

It is easy to forget how integral coal mining is to our country's economy, history and culture. My mother told me that when she was a child in the 1940s, her mother would point out the miners' widows in Morpeth High Street in Northumbria. They were treated with huge respect and sympathy by the community. Once again, this previously familiar national tragedy is in the headlines with five deaths in two mines in recent times, events that will also keep the Health & Safety Executive (HSE) mining inspectorate busy. The HSE website indicates that there are currently 118 mines and 21 licensed underground coalmines employing 3950 personnel (http://www.hse.gov.uk/ mining/how.htm).

The industry is a shadow of its former self. The National Union of Mineworkers estimate that since the 1984 miners strike, 79 pits have closed with the loss of 100 000 jobs (http://www.num.org.uk/page/ History-NumHistory-The-Struggle-Goes-On). The current largest operator is UK Coal with six surface and three deep mines and producing coal for 5% of national electricity production and the domestic market. Making a profit in the industry remains difficult and UK Coal plc, a stock market listed company, made pre-tax losses of £124.6 million in 2010/2011 and £129.1 million in 2009/2010 (http://www.ukcoal.- com/profit-and-loss). Half-year results in 2011 produced a pre-tax profit of £22.1 million.

The high price paid by miners is documented in a roll of honour on the Coalmining History Resources Centre website (http://www.cmhrc.co.uk/site/home/ index.html). It records >164 000 deaths and injuries since 1700.There are also detailed disaster investigation reports, which make sobering reading (http://www.cmhrc.co.uk/site/disasters/index.html). Between 1963 and 1979, there were 10 disasters including the dreadful Aberfan spoil tip collapse in 1966, which engulfed a school and killed 118 children and 28 adults. The others were the Cambrian colliery explosion in 1965 (30 killed), the Michael colliery fire in 1967 (8 killed), an outburst of coal and firedamp at Cynheidre–Pentremawr colliery in 1971 (6 killed), an inrush of water at the Lofthouse colliery in 1973 (7 killed), a rooffall at Seafield colliery in 1973 (5 killed), a cage crash to the bottom of the shaft at Markham colliery in 1973 (18 killed), fire and explosion at Houghton Main colliery in 1975 (6 deaths), derailed train at Bentley colliery in 1978 (7 killed) and an explosion at Golborne colliery in 1979 (10 deaths).

Worldwide, the roll of honour for miners continues to grow and the International Federation of Chemical, Energy, Mine and General Workers' Unions estimates at least 12 000 miners are killed every year although, in many countries, there are no accurately recorded statistics (http://www.icem.org/en/78-ICEMInBrief/4061-As-World-Watches-and-Waits-for-Rescueof-Trapped-Chilean-Miners-What-Can-Prevent-FutureDisasters).

China's mining industry continues to attract attention as it now produces a third of the world's coal. It has a huge domestic demand relying on coal for 70% of its energy production. Data on the China Mining Association website indicates that 2433 miners were killed in 2010 down from 2631 in 2009 (http://www.chinamining.org/News/2011-09-27/1317085273d49910.html).

Mining remains one of the most hazardous occupations known to man.

Source: *Occupational Medicine*, Volume 62, Issue 1, January 2012, Page 16, https://doi.org/10.1093/occmed/kqr175. Copyright © The Author 2011.

Back to school

John Hobson

My medical school year produced four career occupational physicians of whom two are chief medical officers of multinational blue chip companies and one is a professor. Not bad for a year of 160, but perhaps it represents the fading nadir of a golden age. I am sure this number is not unrelated to the fact that at the time we trained, Malcolm Harrington was the professor of occupational medicine in the recently built Institute of Occupational Medicine, and I remember having a whole day dedicated to occupational health, which included an industrial visit. So in an era of declining undergraduate occupational health teaching it was reassuring to be asked to participate in the current undergraduate teaching at Birmingham University, a neat completion of the cycle for me and another of the quartet after a quarter of a century since our qualification. Another Malcolm (Braithwaite) ran the day with military precision and had recruited a cohort of consultants and specialist registrars to assist. Our mission was to supervise small group teaching sessions based on the case of a welder with back pain.

My first surprise was to find that the cavernous pathology museum had disappeared. The rows and rows of specimens in dingy glass cases that I spent hours working among breathing formaldehyde had been replaced with a double-decked layer of smart and functional tutorial rooms. The second surprise was that the first group of 16 students dutifully turned up on time and signed an attendance register. Malcolm's suggested ice breaker was to ask if anyone had experience of working. This was the third surprise. Virtually none of 30 students had ever done any meaningful work apart from the odd waiting on in a restaurant job. Those who had unpaid work experience had taken in it the health service for CV purposes and even these students were in a distinct minority; no porters or cleaners. The nearest to traditional work experience was one student who had worked in a bakery. None of the students had been inside a factory or could identify with anything remotely similar to the photograph of the workshop our fictitious welder worked in. That night on the television there was a feature on the last needle factory in Redditch, where once there were more than a hundred factories producing over 90% of the world's needles. So even in what was once the workshop of the world, it is harder to offer industrial visits, but nevertheless like the teacher who never leaves school, not only do we risk producing a generation of doctors who have not had any occupational health teaching but also we risk a generation of doctors who do not have any meaningful insight into the work of their patients. Even where undergraduate occupational medicine is alive and kicking, the challenge is still greater than we think. Many medical schools don't do any occupational health teaching, and many medical students have no experience of the world of work. As occupational physicians we have a responsibility to rectify both.

Source: *Occupational Medicine*, Volume 63, Issue 1, January 2013, Page 16, https://doi.org/10.1093/occmed/kqs087. Copyright © The Author 2012.

Reprinted by permission of Oxford University Press on behalf of the Society of Occupational Medicine.

Billy Liddell

Anthony Seaton

On my 12th birthday, my father took me (at my request) to watch Liverpool play Arsenal. It was 1950 and my childhood hero was playing on the left wing, his favourite position. He didn't score a goal that day, but I recall the excitement every time he got the ball. I never saw him play again, transferring my interests to rugby, but a tear came to my eye when I heard of his death in 2001.

Billy Liddell's father was a Scots coalminer from near Dunfermline who, like so many in that trade, had no option but to go down the pit on leaving school and so made sure his sons didn't suffer the same fate. When his eldest son, who had shown a precocious aptitude both for football and mathematics, was spotted by Matt Busby as someone who might join him at Liverpool FC, his father insisted that the contract should enable young Billy to continue his accountancy studies. So Billy Liddell pursued both careers simultaneously and it was just as well, for his father died of pneumoconiosis in his 50s leaving his wife with four other children. On £3 a match as a footballer, Billy's accountancy career allowed him enough to bring them down to Liverpool and ensure their futures. He became one of the two most famous footballers of his generation and he and Stanley Matthews were the only ones who represented Great Britain against the Rest of Europe in both those international matches of that decade.

Billy Liddell was a prolific goal scorer, even putting some balls in the net directly from corner kicks. He was respected by his opponents and was the most modest and gentlemanly of men, a Justice of the Peace, a Sunday School teacher and a non-smoker and teetotaller. He had a long career with Liverpool and Scotland and later became bursar of Liverpool University. He fell ill with Parkinson's disease in the 1990s and died in 2001 aged 79. In his obituary, he is said to have suffered latterly from Alzheimer's disease.

Men of my generation will remember the leather football we played with and how heavy it became on wet winter days. Bill Shankly, describing Billy Liddell's scoring ability, said that his headers were like blasts from a gun. On one occasion, he scored with his head from well outside the penalty area. Two decades after I watched him play I found myself seeing patients with neurological damage from professional boxing at the Liverpool Stadium, not far from Anfield. We now know that repeated head trauma can result in both Parkinson's and Alzheimer's disease and, as in the case of Mohammed Ali, you don't need to be knocked senseless. We also know that smoking, whatever its ills, is protective against Parkinson's. Sadly, both father and son seem likely to have died from occupational disease.

Source: *Occupational Medicine*, Volume 65, Issue 1, January 2015, Page 28, https://doi.org/10.1093/occmed/kqu162. Copyright © The Author 2015.

Why I became an occupational physician …

Ann Fingret

In early 1961, I had temporarily abandoned any further attempt to obtain Membership of the Royal College of Physicians as a prelude to a career in psychiatry. I was pregnant and I had a grant from the Imperial Cancer Fund to investigate the diagnosis of breast cancer using radioactive isotopes. Even with this change of direction, a balance between the pressures of academic work and domestic responsibilities was difficult to achieve.

The inevitable happened and I became a partner in a unique general practice in Kentish Town. Income was minimal as the practice, motivated by the strong communist ideals of the senior partners, provided, out of income, the services of a nurse and a social worker. I travelled the area in the family car which was a 1934 Park Ward Bentley. On the practice list was a diverse community of Kentish Town working class (predominantly Irish and Cypriot), Hampstead literati, artists including Sidney Nolan and the London members of the Communist Party. It was a hugely enjoyable experience.

On to the scene came Doreen Miller as a trainee attached to one of the senior partners. She was seeking general practice experience as a prelude to becoming a Medical Officer with Marks and Spencer. Up to this point, I had never heard of Industrial Medicine.

After some months Doreen was asked by Marks and Spencer to undertake locum sessions: we shared the sessions. Suddenly we were working in pristine conditions with no financial constraints in the diagnosis and rehabilitation of the staff. As an in-house medical service, it bore little resemblance to today's practice. Part of our role was to select individuals with perfect health and to reject, without explanation, those who did not meet this target. If staff became ill, referrals were made to private consultants, usually without any reference to their own doctors. I found this difficult to accept but enjoyed the ability to get instant advice for patients.

I also enjoyed dealing with general work-related aspects such as food hygiene and health and safety. The requirement to be a jack of all trades particularly appealed to me and suddenly I had found my niche.

I arranged to see Richard Schilling, a delightful and inspiring man. Following my discussions with him, I realized that this was an exciting and developing field of medicine and I determined to pursue it as a career. I obtained the post of Deputy Head of the Medical Service at John Lewis, acquired my Diploma of Industrial Medicine and became a practitioner in the new specialty of occupational medicine. (It is interesting to note that no additional qualifications were required to become a partner in General Practice or a senior post in occupational medicine.)

I became a member of the Occupational Mental Health Discussion Group: 12 young occupational health physicians exchanging information internationally on stress. This interest largely determined the course of my career.

If not for the advent of Doreen would I have become a psychiatrist? How strange that such happenstance can determine our lives.

Source: *Occupational Medicine*, Volume 57, Issue 5, August 2007, Page 379, https://doi.org/10.1093/occmed/kql129. Copyright © The Author 2007.

Fifty years ago: 'General practice and industrial medicine in the United States'

B.H. Pentney

Given at a meeting of the Association on 3 April 1964.

I am an Appointed Factory Doctor, but it was as a general practitioner that I received a Nuffield Travelling Fellowship for 1963. I had chosen to study the type and range of general practice and the place of the general practitioner in industry. I was also to consider what part the general practitioner could play in a future occupational health service in this country. The tour was started in July 1963 and most of the time was spent in two places—5 weeks in California and 11 weeks in Cincinnati. In North America there is a large and growing body of whole-time industrial physicians, and these are of a high order of knowledge and efficiency. They are the experts. For the greater part they are whole time employees of big industrial organizations. They are responsible for the running of their medical services and research, and set the standard of occupational health throughout the country.

A very comprehensive Workmen's Compensation system is really the basis of the greater part of the work of the general practitioner in industrial medicine, and it is at first sight of immense value in the creation of occupational health systems generally. Unfortunately, during its development the emphasis seems to have altered. The ideals, including fair reimbursement for suffering and loss of earnings, and early rehabilitation, have sometimes been submerged in the processes of preparing a case for presentation to the Accident Commission. The disability will be assessed most carefully—possibly using the standard Packard Thurber system—to achieve some uniformity. Compensation will be awarded strictly in accordance with a standard scale, taking into consideration the patient's age, the exact anatomical site of the lesion, the percentage of loss of movement and expectancy in that man's specific trade. With these tremendously detailed assessments, time is lost and it seemed to me that early and adequate rehabilitation was impeded. I was surprised at the wide range of disabilities accepted as industrial in origin and shocked at the amount of compensation awarded—for example, for bronchitis and coronary disease.

Undoubtedly the general practitioner has an established place in occupational health in the United States. It is, however, fairly limited in its application. Individual and group practitioners provide good casualty and routine examination services for large and small industries.

Although to us it is clearly desirable that all factories should have medical services, occupational health has not yet been completely sold to industry. There industrial medical practitioners dealing mainly with Workmen's Compensation cases have not established free access into plants, and they appear to have little enthusiasm for, or encouragement to be interested in, sick factories. Though splendid and growing centres for environmental studies are available there is much left to be achieved in terms of getting the proprietor or management to want medical services.

Post-graduate training in the speciality is available, but on the whole poorly attended, and it would seem that though this must be made more attractive, the subject of occupational health ought to be a mandatory undergraduate subject.

Source: *Occupational Medicine*, Volume 64, Issue 7, October 2014, Page 489, https://doi.org/10.1093/occmed/kqu033. Copyright © The Author 2014.

Originally from: General practice and industrial medicine in the United States. *Trans Ass Industr Med Offrs* (1964) 14, 89. Available at: *Occup Med (Lond)* 1964;14:89–90. DOI:10.1093/occmed/14.1.89.

Every cloud has a silver lining … even a failed private practice

Nerys Williams

Born in Scotland to an English father and an Irish mother, this man was educated at a Jesuit school before entering Stonyhurst College.

His poor finances led him to seek a respectable job. He studied medicine and spent some time in general practice in Aston near Birmingham. While still young he published several short stories.

He was not, however, an indoor type. During his studies, he spent time as a ship's doctor firstly on a Greenland whaler and then on a voyage up the West African coast. He prepared a paper, published in the *Lancet*, on the diagnosis of leucocythaemia. He then returned to university and completed his doctorate on 'vasomotor changes in tabes dorsalis'.

Having graduated, he joined a practice in Plymouth. But things did not work out and he left to set up his own practice in Portsmouth. He was not successful and had few patients. He used one of his medical teachers at the university, Professor Joseph Bell, to form the basis of his most famous character in short stories. He had worked as ward assistant for Professor Bell and this enabled him to see the man at close quarters. Bell took delight in observing people and said that the walk of a sailor was different than that of a soldier. He was expert at detecting differences in accents and studied the hands to see if there were any calluses or marks which could indicate their job.

Bell said 'all careful teachers have first to show the student how to recognise accurately the case. Recognition depends on accurate and rapid appreciation of small points in which the diseased state differs from the healthy'. Thus, this eminent professor spent time and effort on determining patients' occupations and insisted his students did the same.

From Portsmouth our subject went to Vienna to study ophthalmology. That was also a fiasco and he returned to private practice in Wimpole Street. The same lack of patients occurred again. In his autobiography, he reported that no patients crossed his doorstep. But fate was about to strike. He suffered influenza and was at death's door. He emerged realizing that he could not combine medical and literary careers and so opted for the latter.

His success as a writer of plays and stories was phenomenal but he managed to see military service and it was for this that he was knighted, helped by the fact that the Monarch was a fan. He drove fast cars, spent his life playing golf, flying hot air balloons and airplanes and was into bodybuilding.

Who knows what might have happened if his private practice had been successful. We might have been deprived of Sherlock Holmes and Dr Watson and Arthur Conan Doyle may never have become the household name he is today.

Source: *Occupational Medicine*, Volume 59, Issue 3, May 2009, Page 173, https://doi.org/10.1093/occmed/kqp035. Copyright © The Author 2009.

Reprinted by permission of Oxford University Press on behalf of the Society of Occupational Medicine.

Why I became an occupational physician …

Ralph Ashton

I left school at 16 intending to pursue an interest in bacteriology and obtained a post at a hospital laboratory. Fortunately for me, I met the Professor of Bacteriology at the University of Birmingham who advised that the best route forward would be to study medicine. I applied to the Medical School and was offered a place for 1 year later, providing I obtained a Higher School Certificate. The usual 2 years of study had to be crammed into just one, but I made it and got into the Second Year!

After qualification, house jobs and 2 years National Service in the RAMC, laboratory medicine had lost its appeal. During a short spell in General Practice, I explored other career options and decided Industrial Medicine, as it was then called, was the area for me. This decision was undoubtedly influenced by my upbringing in the Black Country where I lived just 200 m from a drop-forging factory. Among my earliest recollections were exciting visits to the iron foundry where my father was manager. School and later holidays were spent in gas works and I still have a Ministry of Labour and National Service permit enabling me to work as a Gas Company Laboratory Assistant!

I do not recollect any advertised posts in Industrial Medicine so I wrote to many organizations seeking an opening. Responses came from several companies including the Austin Motor Company where Donald Stewart was Chief Medical Officer. He was one of the founders of the Society of Industrial Medical Officers, which later became The Society of Occupational Medicine. Thus, a lifetime in occupational medicine commenced at Longbridge in 1953 in a well-established medical department.

I immediately felt at home in the environment in which I found myself—a large integrated vehicle manufacturing plant, employing at its peak >25 000 workpeople. A wide range of working environments presented many hazards; there was also a large rehabilitation workshop established during World War Two jointly with the Birmingham Accident Hospital, as well as a factory in South Wales where ex-miners disabled by pneumoconiosis, made small metal components and the Austin Model Pedal Car.

Once in post, an attempt at the MRCP convinced me that success was impossible outside hospital. Nevertheless, further study was encouraged and I obtained a DIH. Research opportunities abounded and an MD followed after a 5-year study of impaired working capacity in middle aged men. Other opportunities to gain wider experience included part-time responsibilities in Electricity Generating Stations as well as 'devilling' in medico-legal cases—even providing information about industrial processes for Donald Hunter who stayed with Donald Stewart when he was in Birmingham. The splendid training and experience I received proved invaluable on moving in 1967 to Lucas Industries as Chief Medical Officer.

I have been fortunate to have a professional life full of variety and interest, at home and abroad, and I have never, for one moment, regretted the decision made more than half a century ago.

Source: *Occupational Medicine*, Volume 57, Issue 5, August 2007, Page 366, https://doi.org/10.1093/occmed/kql117. Copyright © The Author 2007.

Reprinted by permission of Oxford University Press on behalf of the Society of Occupational Medicine.

A memorable patient

Mike Gibson

I first met him for a routine, fitness for work medical. He was a 42-year-old non-smoker in a manual but well paid job. Over the next 2 years, I saw little of him as he was fit and well. Then he came to see me to ask about reducing his workload as he was experiencing tiredness and shortness of breath. The ECG performed by his GP had been equivocal and he had been referred to the local cardiologist. I thought the apex beat was more lateral than it should have been and his exercise tolerance was markedly reduced. Pending further investigations, his employer was happy to use him in a less physically demanding role. Some weeks later, he was given a diagnosis of dilated cardiomyopathy with associated cardiac failure. He continued in his protected role for the next few months but, as his exercise tolerance deteriorated, he had to reduce his hours more and more. After 18 months, he had a tertiary referral to an internationally renowned cardiac unit where he was placed on the waiting list for heart transplant. By this time, he was able to manage very light work for only 2h a day.

I reviewed him regularly, for support more than anything specific. He tried to stay upbeat but the situation obviously had a psychological impact on him. He kept his employer and me fully informed of what was going on. After a further year, the cardiac unit offered him a ventricular assist device implanted until such time as a donor heart became available and, as he was still deteriorating, he accepted. He was fitted with a continuous flow device powered by battery through percutaneous wires rather than the alternative pulsatile pump. The battery was attached to a waist harness but he always had to carry a spare battery in a small rucksack. With the device, he was able to continue to work for 2h on 3 separated days a week. He also had to arrange to visit the local A&E Department to tell them what to expect if he collapsed as a result of battery failure or a wire becoming detached. This was the first patient I had seen with this technology and the experience was very interesting. On placing a stethoscope to his chest, no heart sounds were audible—only a continuous hum. Blood pressure was unrecordable by sphygmomanometer as there were no Korotkoff sounds. Unfortunately, I lost touch with him when I retired but there are reports of patients surviving for some years with the device until transplant or even being able to have the device removed after cardiac recovery. But he was the only living patient that I have met who had no pulse.

Source: *Occupational Medicine*, Volume 65, Issue 1, January 2015, Page 53, https://doi.org/10.1093/occmed/kqu087. Copyright © The Author 2015.

The strange case of Irving Selikoff

Anthony Seaton

Irving Selikoff was the leading figure of his time in asbestos research in the United States and a towering presence in occupational medicine. To be a towering presence in occupational medicine in the United States was not as comfortable as it might seem from this side of the Atlantic since the American mindset sees individuals taking sides, democrat or republican, pro- or anti-gun, pro-labour or pro-big business; fences are not there to sit on. So Selikoff was firmly identified with labour and the union movement and attracted opprobrium from industry and its supporters both within and outwith the medical profession. It was whispered that he took money from the unions, though as someone who tried unsuccessfully to do the same thing I would regard it as an indication of his skill as a fundraiser. Most readers will be aware of his pioneering studies of US asbestos workers and his campaigns against the asbestos industry. Fewer will know that he was responsible for the earliest studies of isoniazid as an anti-tuberculosis drug, work that contributed to the later demonstration of the efficacy of triple therapy for that disease.

It is curious that in spite of his notable achievements in medicine, his presidency of the American Thoracic Society and his chair in Mount Sinai, the damaging allegation has been made that he was not properly qualified as a doctor. A search on Google shows some controversy, with statements that he qualified in Scotland, perhaps Edinburgh, and in Middlesex University. What is the truth?

He was born in New York, the son of immigrant Russian Jews. He obtained his bachelor of science degree from Columbia University in 1941 and then went to Glasgow to study medicine at what was then Anderson's College of Medicine and later the medical faculty of Glasgow University but at that time preparing students for the Scottish Triple Qualification through the examining board of the three Scottish Royal Colleges. The war was on and he completed his studies in Australia before returning to take his final examinations. His name appears on the roll of graduates in 1945, when he would have been 30 years old, number 8761. That same year, he returned to the United States and obtained a mysterious MD from Middlesex University, Massachusetts, which was in the throes of closing since the American Medical Association had stopped recognizing its degrees. At the same time, it stopped recognizing qualifications from Anderson's Medical College. Interestingly, both institutions had a reputation for admitting American Jews who found it difficult to gain admission elsewhere. But Selikoff was already embarked on his distinguished career, having completed his medical internships. I am sorry I did not know all this when I knew him since my great grandfather qualified from the same Anderson's College. It is apparent that Selikoff had an early struggle to qualify but qualify he did.

His determination to go to Glasgow and Australia to achieve this was an indication of what was to come. Had he stayed, he would surely have drawn attention to the scandal of mesothelioma then being recognized among the ship workers of Glasgow and first published in Thorax in 1946, 14 years before Chris Wagner's famous paper from South Africa.

Source: *Occupational Medicine*, Volume 60, Issue 1, January 2010, Page 53, https://doi.org/10.1093/occmed/kqp161. Copyright © The Author 2009.

Why I became an occupational physician …

Morris Cooke

Like my predecessors in this series, Malcolm Harrington and David Coggon, I did not initially plan my entry into occupational medicine—indeed it might be said I got in 'by accident' for it was a result of my being invalided from the Royal Army Medical Corps due to illness contracted while serving as dermatologist to Palestine Command in 1946.

The NHS was just starting and my prospects of obtaining a substantive NHS appointment in due course were nil, so my wife Dr Barbara Cooke and I decided to apply for a general practice. We were successful in this for 5 years with my assistantship at the Birmingham Skin Hospital. I had been undertaking several appointments on a part-time basis such as Local Treasury Medical officer when I was approached by chemical manufacturers Albright & Wilson Ltd to do a few sessions, as their doctor was leaving.

I was later approached by their Chief Medical Advisor, Dr John Hughes, and Dr Lloyd Potter, Chief Medical Officer of ICI, and asked to give up general practice and to serve them as occupational physician with a special interest in dermatology. They introduced me to other companies such as Yorkshire Imperial Metals and Alcan and the Skin Hospital were most helpful; I was appointed clinical assistant and given opportunity to continue my interest in occupational dermatology.

I continued personal study at the Institute of Occupational Health where I was appointed to the staff, finally as Honorary Senior Clinical Lecturer. In due course, I was appointed Regional Adviser and to the Department of Industrial Health & Safety at Aston University where I was later appointed part-time Visiting Professor.

I took an increasing interest in the Faculty of Occupational Medicine where I served on the Council and the Specialist Advisory Committee and was an examiner for the Faculty, and also elected President of the Society of Occupational Medicine. At that time, there was consideration as to whether the MRCP should be compulsory before the MFOM. I opposed this view maintaining that the examination for the MFOM including the clinical section should be of a sufficiently high standard on its own. This fortunately was accepted and has proved adequate.

I was appointed FFOM shortly after the Faculty was formed and also CBiol MIBiol, MIEnvSc and MIOSH. Then followed inclusion on the General Medical Council Specialist Register (occupational medicine) and on the Institute of Biology and British Toxicology Society Register of Toxicologists. Research as attached worker at the Medical Research Council Skin Unit on tissue cultures to assess chemical toxicity followed as did election to President of the Royal Society of Medicine Section of Occupational Medicine and Assistant Editorship of the British Journal of Industrial Medicine.

Other appointments continued and a happy and I hope useful career continued. I hope this review and those of my predecessors reassure those interested that there are many ways of entering a specialty even when one initially seems to face insuperable difficulties.

Source: *Occupational Medicine*, Volume 57, Issue 6, September 2007, Page 460, https://doi.org/10.1093/occmed/kql130. Copyright © The Author 2007.

Why I am doing the GCC again

Vanessa Hebditch

'What do you understand by the term "walk the talk"?' was one of the more unconventional questions at my interview for the position of Communication Consultant for the SOM. Having garbled my response and been successfully appointed, I am now literally walking the talk on behalf of the society.

I am just about to embark on my third year as a participant in the Global Corporate Challenge (GCC). It's a workplace health initiative, and this year, as part of the society's team of seven, I'll be joining 180 000 other participants. The aim is to walk 10 000 steps a day. The programme requires you to wear a pedometer for 16 weeks and input your steps into the GCC website. You then go on a virtual team journey around the world and track your team's performance against others and monitor your own achievements.

For the first time, this year I'm really looking forward to it. In Year 1, I was shocked that my usual day involved walking about 4000 steps, so I needed to make some changes to my busy schedule. This was easier for me when I went into the office—I just walked from the mainline train station instead of getting on the tube. When working from home, I had to make an effort to go out at lunchtime. The amazing thing was how walking every day made me 'generally happier'. It also compelled me to think about what I ate. The realization of how much it takes to 'walk-off' a two-finger Kit-Kat made me ask whether I really wanted to eat one. Still, I was delighted to lose 8 kg during the 16-week period.

The initiative is great because it inspires the whole workplace team. I really enjoyed the encouragement I received from my colleagues. Undertaking a personal activity together adds to the team spirit in the office. 'How many steps so far?' I would enquire of Dr John East, the society's medical director, as he entered the office slightly breathless from climbing the stairs. MSN banter reminded us to enter our steps. I felt that if I had a few days when I didn't do my allocated steps I would be letting the whole team down—inspiration for me to make them up at the weekend.

For me, the success of the initiative has been in Year 2. After the first year, I found that I quickly reverted to my old ways. You don't need to be Sherlock Holmes to guess that I lost the fitness and other benefits and regained the weight. The second year I incorporated other activities as well as walking and started going to the gym. This time I have sustained it. I'd recommend any company to get their staff involved. The GCC website (www.gettheworldmoving.com) gives information on the benefits for the individual and for the employer. A big personal thank you to Dr David Batman, formerly from Nestlé, who has supported the society each year and enabled us to enter a team.

Source: *Occupational Medicine*, Volume 62, Issue 4, 4 June 2012, Page 307, https://doi.org/10.1093/occmed/kqs059. Copyright © The Author 2012.

Fifty years ago: 'The appointed factory doctor'

Anon

It is now generally accepted that as a nation we have too few doctors, and this fact is frequently emphasized when expansion of occupational health services is under discussion. The appointed factory doctor system is thought by some to provide a possible solution to this difficulty. Here, it is urged, is a body of men who between them cover the whole of the country, and who are already working in industry, which could be used as a nucleus of a nation-wide occupational health service, without making demands on our medical manpower which could not be met without starving the curative health services.

Most of the 1700 A.F.D.'s are general practitioners whose main professional interests are in domiciliary medicine; for them the appointment can become an interesting but minor sideline. Increasingly the full-time industrial medical officer has entered the picture, but he is restricted to the examination of young persons and employees covered by special regulations. The volume of work performed by A.F.D.'s in 1963, to take a typical recent year, raises some interesting questions. 51 9705 juveniles were examined; all but 21 167 were passed without conditions affecting their employability. Only 1449 juveniles were completely rejected for employment, and of these a disproportionate number were girls. Over half the 848 females rejected suffered from pediculosis, and 212 of the 601 boys suffered from visual refractive errors. Both these conditions are quickly and eminently remediable. Their very existence as causes of rejection raises the question of the true functions and the proper use of the system of examining juveniles.

A further 358 904 examinations were performed in 1963 under the special regulations governing hazardous occupations, and they resulted in 999 suspensions from work. The low proportion of suspensions is almost certainly attributable to the efficiency of the physical control measures in force in these processes. In some trades, the control is obviously so efficient that the question arises whether the continuation of medical examinations is justified, and whether environmental control measures alone are now all that are needed.

It should not be forgotten that by far the greater part of the total work of the A.F.D. system is done in the thickly populated, highly industrialized conurbations. These unlovely areas have other pressing problems of medical care, morbidity is higher in such areas, they have fewer general practitioners and their hospitals attract fewer junior staff, so that supplemental staffing by local family doctors is often necessary. The medical resources of such towns are already severely overstrained and relatively small extra burdens, such as the work of the A.F.D., always mean robbing Peter to pay Paul.

The role and functions of the A.F.D. are, for this and other reasons, in need of re-appraisal and re-definition. Some of his existing duties seem to be superfluous, whilst others are not performed effectively. If the job is to be made more precise, it will be necessary to ensure that the appointees have not only the knowledge and training, but also the time to perform their new duties adequately. This latter factor is easily estimable and will become increasingly important as the medical man-power crisis deepens during the present decade.

Source: *Occupational Medicine*, Volume 64, Issue 7, October 2014, Page 529, https://doi.org/10.1093/occmed/kqu035. Copyright © The Author 2014.

Originally from: The appointed factory doctor. *Trans Ass Industr Med Offrs* (1964) 14, 65. Available at: *Occup Med (Lond)* 1964;14:65. DOI:10.1093/occmed/14.1.65.

Mesothelioma

John Hobson

There are three cases of mesothelioma that stand out in my mind during my career as an occupational physician. The first was a lagger I encountered whilst I was a trainee working for a power generation company. I visited him at home to talk about ill health retirement, the cooling towers of the power station he had lagged 20 years beforehand looming over his back garden. Only in his mid-forties, he was bewildered, and I came away feeling hopeless and helpless. I had seen one or two cases whilst working on a chest ward but this was palpably a terrible occupational disease. The second memorable case was 20 years later: a very fit and healthy manager in his late forties who had worked in the same factory as I had for a similar length of time. The majority of his working life had been in offices and not the shop-floor. He hadn't worked in departments where we knew there was an asbestos legacy and where I had been keeping an eye on the toll of mesothelioma cases slowly mounting in long retired workers. It was difficult to understand how this manager had contracted the condition and worrying to think that his relevant exposure was probably the general factory environment.

The ever increasing death rate of mesothelioma in the UK is frightening. In 1968 there were 153 deaths. In 2009 there were 2321 deaths from the condition, only a few hundred more than people claiming disablement benefit. The median time from diagnosis to death remains stubbornly fixed at 18 months. In males, death rates show an almost perfect 10-fold increase with increasing age: one death per 10 million in 30-year-olds, one death per million in 40-year-olds, one death per 100 000 in 50-year-olds, one death per 10 000 in 60-year-olds and approaching one death per 1000 in 70-year-olds. Those who die are those who worked in certain occupations. This has shifted from primary users, such as those who manufactured and made products with asbestos and classical occupations such as shipbuilding, to secondary users or those who come into contact with asbestos as part of their work and specifically those in construction and craft trades, plumbers, carpenters, and electricians. Male deaths are estimated to peak in 2016, but this does not look certain from the graphs.

The third case rang me in 2011. He had heard a scratching noise in his chest when he was in bed. He rang me because he knew my speciality but also because he wanted me to provide a witness statement. Did I remember the underground passageway between the medical school and the hospital 30 years ago? The overhead pipes, the crumbling lagging, the number of times we had used it, the adjacent pigeon holes and seating area where we often met and had a chat and a coffee as medical students. He died aged 50, 7 months after the phone call. I still have the voicemail.

Source: *Occupational Medicine*, Volume 63, Issue 2, March 2013, Page 108, https://doi.org/10.1093/occmed/kqs045. Copyright © The Author 2013.

Why I became an occupational physician ...

Ian S. Symington

It was in the 1970s that I first had experience of dealing with work-related disease. I was climbing the National Health Service career ladder towards becoming a consultant physician and spent 2 years in Glasgow Western Infirmary's respiratory unit. Unfortunately, there was little which could be done therapeutically for the majority of the work-related respiratory disease I saw. But one morning at the asthma clinic, a patient attended with features of 'late onset' asthma. She told me about her work in a food factory where dried packet soups were produced and how she used a compressed air jet to clean the soup dust from the machinery thus releasing clouds of dust into her lungs. Investigations followed, using samples of the soup ingredients as a basis for immunological skin testing and inhalation challenge tests. These confirmed an occupational cause and incriminated mushroom dust as the key allergen. Visits to the factory led to the discovery of others with similar symptoms and liaison with the company's doctor facilitated environmental improvements [1]. Was this patient—'the case who changed my career'? Well, she certainly stimulated me to consider how health gains could be achieved through environmental changes rather than conventional therapeutics.

Some other work-related health projects then came my way, including a study of firemen's health and smoke inhalation. This led to liaison with Eric Blackadder, the head of the Employment Medical Advisory Service (EMAS) in Scotland. His enthusiastic approach was quite inspirational and EMAS's range of activities at that time appeared impressive. He had just returned from a Scotland-wide study of distillery workers which established the prevalence of malt workers lung, and this project had allegedly involved sampling a wee dram at each establishment. It became clear that there were doctors who actually worked full-time in this field and, sensing my interest, Eric asked me to consider becoming an occupational physician.

I did eventually apply for an EMAS post but the Civil Service application form had a complete page entitled 'previous relevant experience'. As I had no direct experience, I filled the space with work activities during medical school vacations. These included construction work in tunnels, catering, driving trucks, labouring in sub-zero refrigeration plants, functioning as a docker and, most stressful of all, instructing people how to drive. During the interview chaired by Suzette Gauvain, with Ken Duncan and Peter Taylor providing a formidable team, the questions focussed mainly on my experiences in these environments and I demonstrated at least some knowledge of the world of work.

And so I was successful in being recruited to the ideal job with 50% of my time devoted to practical EMAS service activity and 50% to teaching and research in the Department of Community and Occupational Medicine in the University of Dundee, with Professors Alex Mair and Bill Taylor. I never looked back and I consider myself most fortunate to have had the support of these distinguished mentors, along with many others, during these early years.

Reference

1. **Symington IS, Kerr JW, McLean DA.** Type 1 allergy in mushroom soup processors. *Clin Allergy* 1981;**11**:43–47.

Source: *Occupational Medicine*, Volume 57, Issue 6, September 2007, Page 390, https://doi.org/10.1093/occmed/kql159. Copyright © The Author 2007.

Sydney 2000

Mike McKiernan

The athletic shadow of Millennium Man with his boomerang bursting limbs strides majestically over the city, its five white Olympic rings and the iconic Opera House—a motif echoed in the smoke plume of his torch and repeated on his legs. The blue background mimicking sea and sky is composed of the names of all the competing nations. Sydney 2000 'the athletes' Games' has been acknowledged by many as the best Olympics ever.

Captain Robert Dover opened the first Olimpicks in the Cotswold town of Chipping Campden (1612); Dr William Brookes launched the first Olympian Games in Much Wenlock, Shropshire (1850); and Baron Pierre de Coubertin inaugurated the first Modern Games in Athens (1896). London 2012 will be the XXX Olympiad and will feature 10 500 athletes representing 200 countries in 26 sports. There will be 6250 anti-doping samples, 375 doctors, 150 nurses, 200 000 pairs of gloves and 150 000 condoms. The Games will cost £11.3 billion; be watched by 10 million spectators; and be reported on by 21 000 media personnel. Organizers hope that the Games will leave a 'sustainable legacy of national benefits in culture, sport, volunteering, business and tourism'. Sadly Captain Dover's shin-kicking competition is no longer an Olympic sport.

Source: *Occupational Medicine*, Volume 62, Issue 5, 5 July 2012, Page 330, https://doi.org/10.1093/occmed/kqs076. Copyright © The Author 2012.

Tales of Kieran: The occupational physician's odyssey 4—Vanadium

J.A. Hunter

Kieran invited me to his college for dinner recently, and after he had proudly given me a guided tour of how academia lives, we had a very pleasant meal and some excellent wine. We took port with another Fellow from St Arrhenius currently doing some experimental work at the local power station. In these energy-conscious times, they have been trying to burn low-grade Venezuelan bitumen because nobody else wants it and it is very cheap. Kieran became very excited about this and the two were soon engrossed in deep conversation. I was happily dozing off when Kieran suddenly demanded my 'expert opinion'.

'You are a proper physician', he said. 'You must know all about vanadium pneumonitis?' Somewhat taken aback and wondering how much of the conversation I had slept through, I confessed rather shamefully that I did not have the foggiest and, feeling slightly embarrassed in such cerebral surroundings, made my apologies and then for home.

Intrigued despite my soporific state, I consulted my medical textbooks at home but without much success. It was not until the next day in the hospital library that I managed to unearth any reference to vanadium at all. I discovered that Venezuelan oil derives from sea creatures particularly rich in vanadium. The oil burns to leave a large ash residue, exposure to which causes vanadium poisoning and a very bizarre collection of clinical findings. Good stuff this occupational medicine, I thought!

A few days later, while sat in the mess, I overheard a couple of juniors mention 'the case with classical vanadium poisoning currently on the wards'. Never one to dismiss a coincidence, I immediately telephoned Kieran, to be told by his secretary that unfortunately he had been admitted to hospital with a chest complaint. Putting two and two together, I dashed up to the chest ward. Sure enough, there he was in a side room, oxygen mask on and somewhat red-faced when he saw me enter. Refusing to even open his mouth to me, he immediately pressed the buzzer and had sister usher me out whilst reminding her of medical confidentiality.

Determined to get to the bottom of this one, I hit on the brainwave of ringing the chemist we had taken port with at the college a few nights previously. I was a little surprised at the reception I got.

'I hope you are nothing to do with that lunatic!' he raved most unacademically down the telephone. 'He almost managed to black out the whole of Linfordshire AND we nearly lost our contract with the power company.' I assured him as best I could that I only knew Kieran as an occasional acquaintance, and he reluctantly continued. 'Well, he absolutely insisted on entering the boiler to take samples for vanadium to make sure there was no health hazard when we entered. I wouldn't mind but we had all been in quite happily without any adverse effects and the power station wanted to start the boiler up again. But no, he insisted—"protecting university staff", he called it. And then he had the audacity of threatening to call the unions if he was not allowed access. He was in there for over six hours with his sampling apparatus because each time he came out they tried to take the scaffolding down.'

'But why didn't he wear a mask?' I asked timorously.

'He did, but they don't work very well with beards. Serves him right, if you ask me. The man's a nutter.'

I planned out my next move carefully. Having found some tame medical students, I burst into Kieran's room after sister accepted it was all in aid of medical education. 'And this patient has very kindly agreed to demonstrate the pathognomic sign of acute vanadium poisoning.' Kieran knew when he was beaten and obliged. The students presumably thought this was simply a rude, unco-operative patient, but that bright green tongue said it all!

Source: *Occupational Medicine,* Volume 52, Issue 6, September 2002, Page 359, https://doi.org/10.1093/occmed/52.6.359. Copyright © Society of Occupational Medicine 2002.

Directly read

John Challenor

Occupational physicians share a common medical and surgical background. All of us have passed through medical school and trained to a greater or lesser extent in several medical and surgical specialties. While our shared experience is often subsumed by our more recent practice in occupational medicine, it takes little to refresh the memories of those student days and training posts. Recently, while browsing the shelves of my favourite book seller, I came across a delightful little book that evoked many memories. The author Gabriel Weston is a part-time ear, nose, and throat surgeon in London and an English graduate of Edinburgh University and has produced a charming and readable selection of short stories.

Very often, when doctors turn their hand to writing their writer's cramp is reflected in their prose. Not so in the case of Weston's collection of succulent vignettes, which have been gleaned from her experience as a medical student and young surgeon. This small book of only 181 pages naturally dissects into 14 chapters of comfortable volume that most readers will find both appetizing and digestible. Even those with busy lives and less time for the self-indulgence of enjoying a good read will find pleasurable reminiscences in the pages of this book.

It is surprising that descriptions of events in a junior doctor's life still hold such fascination. Why this should be is clearly grounded in the author's acuteness of perception and her skill in constructing enticing story lines: a combination of two distinct but synergistic skills—the writer's craft and the surgeon's craft. Death, beauty, hierarchy, territory and ambition are headings that give clues to the content of the chapters. The excision of a submandibular gland by the author when she was a junior cannot fail to stir memories of one's own junior surgical house jobs. 'I have tied off Wharton's duct and the gland is hanging from its pedicle'. 'Cut it, come on', goads the chief. 'Cut it! What are you, chicken? Cut it, chicken!' The facial artery is severed and 'blood sprays a foot across the room'. 'I feel slow, clumsy, dangerous and ashamed'.

Occupational physicians working in the health care sector may need reminding that junior staff as well as more senior colleagues even today experience some of the attitudes, prejudices and pressures described by Dr Weston. On the other hand, some workers allege harassment and bullying when what they are experiencing is fair but firm management; a reminder that we have to have our wits about us if we are to provide sound advice to all strata of workers.

Here is a book that is affordable, short and beautifully written. Undeniably contemporary, it has the makings of a classic. My copy will sit next to 'A Fortunate Man' and 'The Story of San Michele'. Buy this book for those who are thinking of a career in medicine as it will paint a picture of what life was like and is often still like. Read it during those rare quiet moments and it will make you smile.

Source: *Occupational Medicine*, Volume 60, Issue 1, January 2010, Page 20, https://doi.org/10.1093/occmed/kqp153. Copyright © The Author 2009.

Why I became an occupational physician …

Peter Harries

I was lucky enough to be a student at The London Hospital when Donald Hunter was teaching and Director of the Department for Research in Industrial Medicine at 'The London'. He was inspiring, hyperactive and nobody slept in his lectures! He always started his lectures with the precise words he had ended the last. He was then putting the finishing touches to the first edition of his masterpiece *The Diseases of Occupations*. This must be the finest historical account of occupational medicine. His department included many who were, or became, distinguished occupational physicians. Among them were Ian McLaughlin, John Bonnell, Lesley Bidstrup and George Kazantzis.

During my Naval National Service, I tried to deal with the effects of excessive noise in the engine room of a frigate, but with little success. I was then appointed to the Occupational Health Department of Devonport Dockyard. While there I sat the Diploma in Industrial Medicine and wrote answers on the findings I had made on medical examinations on asbestos workers and others in the dockyard. These answers were picked up at the oral exam by Richard Schilling who wrote to the Medical Director of the Royal Navy advising that a study of the extent of the problem should be undertaken. This resulted in my appointment as Director of the study on behalf of the Ministry of Defence and the Medical Research Council (MRC). Richard Schilling played a big supervisory role together with John Gilson and his colleagues, John Cotes, Peter Oldham and Vernon Timbrell at the MRC Pneumoconiosis Unit Penarth. The results were published as my MD thesis and Schilling and Gilson recommended that the study be replicated in Portsmouth, Chatham and Rosyth Dockyards. This involved another 6 years work and the total study population was 40 000 with 84% compliance. The results of the studies resulted in widespread changes in working practices for all dockyards, many of which were introduced during the Devonport study.

At this stage, I wanted a change and, again, Richard Schilling advised me to accept the post of Chief Medical Officer to Rank Hovis McDougall, flour miller, bakers and food manufacturers. This was another challenging job which was very rewarding.

Donald Hunter whetted my appetite for occupational medicine but it was Richard Schilling who really inspired me and guided my career.

Source: *Occupational Medicine*, Volume 57, Issue 7, October 2007, Page 537, https://doi.org/10.1093/occmed/kql131. Copyright © The Author 2007.

A leaky vessel

Richard Colman

Arthur works on a production line making chemical fertilizers. He works with six other colleagues in an enclosure containing three chemical vessels. Arthur is referred to occupational health because of a skin rash which he feels is due to a toxic substance leaking from one of the vessels. Arthur has had skin problems previously and when working for another company was off work for four months. At the consultation the exact cause of the problem is uncertain but it is possible that he has developed a recognized condition consistent with exposure to a noxious substance. No other workers are experiencing the same problem. Arthur feels management have not taken his concerns seriously; they see him as a bit of a moaner; he insisted on a referral to occupational health because he didn't want to go of sick again and he says that 'companies are not supposed to make their employees ill'.

The occupational physician reports a problem and expresses concerns that one of the vessels may be leaking a toxic substance. Management have a procedure to risk assess and evaluate the competency of the vessel but the substance is hard to measure directly so the objectivity of the assessment is limited. Management interpret the evidence as equivocal and non-conclusive. A problem with the vessel is not acknowledged. Nonetheless, Arthur is moved to a different environment fortunately with no financial detriment.

Meanwhile management seek the possibility of screening out potentially vulnerable employees at the pre-appointment stage. The occupational physician reports this would be unnecessarily discriminatory on the grounds that skin problems are common and the adverse reaction relatively rare. Six months later another worker presents with a skin problem and he considers it due to the same leaky vessel as did Arthur. This time the employee is in danger of losing his job as redeployment will be difficult.

Management don't like the occupational health advice to fix the problem. Their internal assessment has exonerated them of the problem and they consider the employee has an alternative agenda. However the occupational physician feels there still may be a work-related condition and so visits the site and talks to employees. They raise a concern about the vessel but are not sufficiently affected to take it further. Others have moved out as soon as possible. The occupational physician reviews the risk assessment and questions the appropriateness of the assessment and its interpretation. It confirms concerns about exposure to a toxic influence. On meeting his own line manager the occupational physician is told of complaints about his 'one-sided' reports. They have no evidence for a leaking vessel or toxic substance.

Now replace the leaky vessel with 'line manager', skin disorder with 'anxiety and depression', vulnerability with 'anxious personality', risk assessment with 'stress risk assessment', toxic with 'bullying management style'. The occupational physician is told he should not infer there is a 'problem manager'; he should not criticize management and only see one side and by the way the contract might be in jeopardy.

Source: *Occupational Medicine*, Volume 62, Issue 6, September 2012, Page 465, https://doi.org/10.1093/occmed/kqs101. Copyright © The Author 2012.

Reprinted by permission of Oxford University Press on behalf of the Society of Occupational Medicine.

Fifty years ago: 'Parameters of occupational health in America'

H. Beric Wright

Based on a paper read to the Association on 3 April 1964 following a seven week visit to the USA in the Autumn of 1963.

The distribution of in-plant services is much the same as it is in this country, most large firms having a medical department with full-time doctors and many more using full-time nurses and part-time local practitioners. The Industrial Medical Association in America has 3000 members of whom about one-third are full-time, but this figure probably includes people in university departments. About 400 of them are Board-certified specialists.

Formerly there were 43 University departments in the USA and Canada teaching industrial medicine. It was realized that many of these were below the necessary standard and a system of inspection and reporting was instituted so that there are now about 15 Universities which run courses for doctors and industrial hygienists.

Probably unfortunately, the US specialist boards require a 3-year course for a Master's degree, so that although a steady stream of hygienists is produced, each course seems to attract relatively few doctors. Indeed, the length of the course and the fact that salaries in industry compare on the whole unfavourably with those that can be earned in private practice, mean that industrial medicine is not on the whole attracting the right people. There is some anxiety about the fact that it is becoming rather a depressed speciality.

To conclude

All is not gold that glitters, either in America or anywhere else. Basically both the incidence and the efficacy of occupational health in the USA are much the same as here, and the problems are the same—how to get small- and medium-sized firms to 'do the right thing'; how to attract and train the right doctors, and how far should compulsory legislation go towards enforcing reasonable standards? Americans have more money for research, better physical conditions in factories and offices (although there are also plenty of bad 'railway arch' workshops, totally unsupervised), but the universities tend to be disappointing and doctors in industry are in short supply. There do seem to be two overwhelming advantages in America—the willingness of central government to spend money on long-term research and the availability, through insurance companies and some States, of virtually free occupational hygiene advice. I started by saying that America is a large and disparate country. I found that it became more exciting as I got further west, until I finally left my heart in San Francisco. But apart from charm and atmosphere, the west coast is doing new things, from the Kaiser small plant service and their socialized Permanente plan, through two group practices doing nothing but industrial medicine, to the occupational health department at Washington University in Seattle, which is supported by a tax on industry matched by a contribution from the unions. This State also has a comprehensive and compulsory industrial insurance scheme. The east coast I found less dynamic and prone to worshipping its own image and past achievement, but it too will do new things and those two grand old men of industrial medicine, Kehoe in Cincinnati and Ted Hatch in Pittsburgh, are now studying health rather than disease. Hatch is trying to find out what contribution work makes to the falling off of capacity with age.

Source: *Occupational Medicine*, Volume 64, Issue 8, December 2014, Page 648, https://doi.org/10.1093/occmed/kqu034. Copyright © The Author 2014.

Originally from: Parameters of occupational health in America. *Trans Ass Industr Med Offrs* (1964) 14, 91. Available at: *Occup Med (Lond)* 1964;14:91–95. DOI:10.1093/ occmed/14.1.91.

More genetics for medical students?

Anthony Seaton

Calls come regularly from people wishing to expand the curriculum and from others wishing to simplify it lest students suffer from an overload, so those at the sharp end wonder what to drop if the latest enthusiasm is introduced. The House of Lords has called for more training of doctors in genetics in order to fit them for 21st century practice—personalized medicine, genetic risk identification and so on. Juxtaposed in the media are reports of the pension crisis, economic collapse, climate change and diminishing energy resources.

The health of the public presents some serious challenges to doctors and the National Health Service (NHS). These include such conditions as diabetes, asthma, obesity and alcohol-related illness, all rising in prevalence and thus related to environmental rather than genetic change. The challenge is to identify the risk factors and to reduce them, a neglected area of research, but the fact that such research investment pays off is shown by studies of heart disease. We also have the problem of increasing numbers of physically or mentally disabled old people, a consequence of an improved healthier environment over 50 years. The challenge is again to find modifiable factors in the environment that increase or reduce the risk of such conditions as Parkinson's and Alzheimer's diseases. Alongside these, climate change and the crisis of capitalism will bring increasing pressure of immigration to less affected nations such as ours; the economic environment of our children and grandchildren will revert to one such as we endured in the 1940s and 1950s. The provision of the welfare state is already less all embracing and pensions are becoming increasingly expensive. The NHS will struggle to maintain its level of funding. Will the new genetics help us solve these problems?

There is in medical research a disparity between the resources devoted to detecting and measuring risk factors for common disabling diseases and those devoted to genetics, which accepts that disease will occur and hopes to find a cure. Advances in understanding genetics are relevant to understanding microorganisms, allow us to develop vaccines and other treatments and will be important in understanding why one person falls ill and another does not. They may be of benefit to the pharmaceutical industry but are likely to impose an unacceptable extra cost on the NHS. Illness is essentially a failure of adaptation to an individual's environment, owing partly to genetic make-up and partly to environmental factors. We have the genes we were born with and we should aim to help our patients readapt to the environment that is most conducive to a healthy life. Medical advances are a necessary part of this adaptation, but any increase in genetic teaching of doctors must be balanced by teaching of nutritional and lifestyle risk factors. Our genes have evolved under external pressures; their expression is modulated by alterations in the environment in which we live. By all means, teach genetics but let us not forget the environment.

Source: *Occupational Medicine*, Volume 60, Issue 8, December 2010, Page 667, https://doi.org/10.1093/occmed/kqq161. Copyright © The Author 2010.
Reprinted by permission of Oxford University Press on behalf of the Society of Occupational Medicine.

Why I became an occupational physician …

Monty Brill

My undergraduate course at Glasgow in the early 1950s was the first to be extended to 6 years and among many changes the Public Health module had become Social Medicine. I vaguely remember being given an introduction to Industrial Health—no doubt due to the influence of Andrew Meiklejohn (notable for his contribution to dust diseases in miners). I was also aware that the Glasgow Faculty (now College) of Physicians and Surgeons granted a DIH and thought one day I might look into that.

A decade later, as a junior partner in general practice in East London with a young family to support, the need to augment my income was pressing. I managed to fill most afternoons with additional work in Maternal and Child Welfare and, most importantly as it turned out, I was appointed the doctor to an engineering company making small parts for motorcar manufacturers. Management expectations were that I would weed out the sick and lazy at preemployment and push absentees back to full work. Soon after starting, I was presented with a man who had a nasal perforation from working in the chrome plating shop and several others with dermatitis employed in machining areas. Venturing into the plant, I found they were manufacturing the outer casings of spark plugs. Metal bars were machined into shells, degreased in trichlorethylene and then shaken upright and sorted.

Two patients in the practice were working in a nearby Lead Battery factory and described their working conditions. At around the same period, Desmond Terry gave a BMA lunchtime talk on asbestos. Here was a group of industrial diseases that I knew little about and felt I should know more. Also at that time, I came across Donald Hunter's Pelican, Health in Industry.

I continued to work now as sole principal and grew enthusiastic over forming a group practice with ancillary staff which is now the NHS norm. My efforts to promote this with local colleagues failed and, having written a couple of articles on the subject, I wanted to develop my options in other directions.

I enrolled in the part time Society of Apothecaries course that would lead to the DIH. The lecturers included AIG McLaughlin, Bob Murray and Ron Owen. Ron made sure that at the end of the course we were all admitted into membership of the SOM.

Walking up the steps of the recently completed Lasdun Royal College building to my first SOM Autumn meeting, I was acutely aware that there would not be a single person I would know. Entering the hall, I was approached by the President, Andrew Raffle, who welcomed me and introduced me to a number of other members.

The meeting was enjoyable and instructive but most of all I felt very comfortable in the realization that I would have colleagues to turn to for support.

Within the year, I took up a full-time post as a medical officer in Ford Motor Company where I remained until I retired in 1992.

Source: *Occupational Medicine*, Volume 57, Issue 8, December 2007, Page 614, https://doi.org/10.1093/occmed/kql140. Copyright © The Author 2007.

Reprinted by permission of Oxford University Press on behalf of the Society of Occupational Medicine.

Charmed to be sure

Arthur Eakins

The countryman is perhaps a more simple trusting soul, but with a degree of cunning, quite different from his counterpart used to a more comfortable urban life of convenience. This contrast became evident one dark winter's night in the west of Northern Ireland. The Ballygawley roundabout is a well-known landmark, dividing the Province into east and west. To the west, it is pure farming country where science has not fully arrived to some living in this land. There is a belief in fairies and charms; farmers are loath to disturb fairy mounds and the phase of the moon needs to be ascertained as it could be testing providence to take important decisions at the full moon.

Having seen a long line of appointments all day, my last man came in and sat down carefully. He was a well-built man with a large ruddy face. His high colour I suspected was due to a mixture of fresh air and Guinness. It was six weeks since he had been able to give service to his employers, and they not unreasonably wished to know if and when he was likely to resume work. After a short discourse on the weather, he was questioned on his absence due to illness. Sick certificates showed haemorrhoids, which was confirmed by the patient as 'terrible poiles'. Further confirmation of his condition followed. He dressed and pulled on a heavy winter greatcoat.

On treatment for his distressing condition, he volunteered that he was relying on a charm. Seeing my astonishment, he became somewhat indignant at my disbelief and the charm was produced from his greatcoat. It consisted of a piece of brown paper screwed up and held together by Sellotape. When I told him that there was nothing inside and I threatened to unravel it, he became quite animated. If the paper was unravelled, properties of the charm would be lost and his 'poiles' would remain. No amount of argument was going to alter his mind, so we agreed to differ.

Purveyors of charms are usually old ladies, who have the powers to make up charms, for a modest fee. Thyme, chamomile, and cockspur grass are sometimes used as the basis of treatment for a variety of conditions. Copper bangles are credited with curative powers, and worn to reduce arthritic symptoms by a surprising spectrum of the population. Liaison by the occupational physician with the general practitioner in such cases may bring about a more dynamic mode of treatment, giving ease to both employer and employee. One wonders however, if brown paper and Sellotape will ever make it into the NICE therapeutic lexicon for gastrointestinal conditions?

Source: *Occupational Medicine*, Volume 62, Issue 8, December 2012, Page 668, https://doi.org/10.1093/occmed/kqs150. Copyright © The Author 2012.

Reprinted by permission of Oxford University Press on behalf of the Society of Occupational Medicine.

A practical demonstration of Boyle's Law

Mike Gibson

Over 30 years ago I was working in the Altitude Research Section of the (now sadly defunct) Royal Air Force Institute of Aviation Medicine. At the time we were testing the prototype of a respirator intended to protect aircrew from nuclear, biological and chemical agents. This respirator was designed to be part of the normal oxygen delivery system required to prevent hypoxia in flight. We needed to confirm that the respirator still delivered enough oxygen to the aircrew during a rapid decompression in the event of a failure of the aircraft pressurization system.

The test was carried out in the high-performance decompression chamber. Because of the risk of loss of consciousness, I was placed in a supine posture on a standard medical examination couch, with a bicycle ergometer mounted at the foot end so that the normal workload of piloting an aircraft could be simulated. I was comfortable in the respirator, which I had worn many times before. A probe from a respiratory mass spectrometer was placed in the oronasal facemask to monitor breath by breath oxygen tensions. The chamber was taken gently up to a simulated base altitude of 8000 feet. I started pedalling at a predetermined rate and load and, when the measurements indicated a steady state, the countdown started for a rapid decompression in less than a second to a simulated altitude of 33 000 feet. As usual, I exhaled in the second or two before decompression to prevent air embolism as lung gases expanded.

There was the usual 'bang' and the instant formation of a cold mist. But what I was not prepared for was suddenly being lifted 2–3 inches into the air as the air in the padding below the fake leather cover of the examination couch expanded approximately 4-fold. I then gently subsided as the outlet valves on the sides of the couch let the air out with a loud and prolonged, raspberry noise. It was certainly a different way of demonstrating Boyle's Law, first published in 1662, which states that the absolute pressure and volume of a given mass of confined gas are inversely proportional if the temperature remains constant, i.e. $P1\ V1 = P2\ V2$.

Source: *Occupational Medicine*, Volume 65, Issue 2, March 2015, Page 109, https://doi.org/10.1093/occmed/kqu101. Copyright © The Author 2015.

Reprinted by permission of Oxford University Press on behalf of the Society of Occupational Medicine.

Lest we forget

John Hobson

It's six thirty in the morning but the city is already awake and on its way to work. I bump and rattle over the cobbled streets that lead through the old docks before entering the industrial flatland that stretches from Antwerp to Rotterdam. Cars race past me on their way to work as we drive through a never-ending vista of docked ships and cranes, grain silos and train marshalling yards, oil refineries and chemical plants. Out of the pre-dawn darkness my particular refinery emerges, radiant and resplendent like an uninhabited mini-Manhattan. Others can be seen in the distance, adorned with white lights, red lights up their stacks and crowned by defiant gas flares high in the night sky. It's a sight that still excites, even after a quarter century of industrial practice and its good being part of it. I'm here to do 80 asbestos medicals on some of the four and a half thousand contractors drafted in for the refinery's shutdown. Some of the medicals are conducted in English, others in French but the majority through an interpreter. The contractors I see are mainly eastern European, something increasingly familiar in the last 10 years, whether it is chicken factory workers in East Anglia or pottery workers in the West Midlands. The manager tells me that the Czechs and Slovaks are more reliable than the UK workers who often disappear before the contract ends. He laments all the older workers who have contracted lymphoma and malignancies which he attributes to oil and chemical exposures.

At least the environmental and engineering controls are better now he says. Before each round of medicals I hear the toolbox safety talk in English and Czech. In the afternoon I go to the Magritte museum in Brussels. Walking through the city it strikes me how we are actually governed from this place. A strange concept for the UK, only a couple of hours drive away but somehow still on the margin of Europe. The politicians of Brussels are probably the reason why I am carrying out these medicals but also why health and safety controls and practices have improved. It is easy to overlook the good that comes from Belgium; it is less easy to ignore the bad that has happened in Belgium. Half an hour down the road, 300 000 European men fought each other at Waterloo and another hour to the west a hundred years later, the same number of British and Commonwealth men died defending the Ypres Salient. In Ieper, the massive Menin Gate is inscribed with 55 000 names of the 90 000 soldiers who were never found or identified. There was not enough space and the other 35 000 names are inscribed at Tyne Cot 10km away. Named after the first aid post that still remains and surrounded by row after row after row of white grave stones, Tyne Cot is the largest war cemetery in the world. Wandering amongst the headstones it is hard to find any inscribed with names. 'Lest we forget.'

Source: *Occupational Medicine*, Volume 64, Issue 1, January 2014, Page 30, https://doi.org/10.1093/occmed/kqt128. Copyright © The Author 2013.

Why I became an occupational physician …

Andy Slovak

On June 27 1948, I arrived at Dover on M.V. King Albert, aged 2¼, an asylum-seeking alien ahead of my parents yet to smuggle themselves out of Czechoslovakia. It was a rude shock for them to arrive with nothing in austere post-war England. Unable to teach without UK qualifications, my father took jobs that the indigenous population would not and became a foreman in a Hammersmith cement works lugging 2 cwt cement bags. I did my first industrial visit with him aged 3½ and was struck vividly by the dust which coated everything and the sheer grinding physical effort involved. After a couple of years, he got a job as an industrial chemist (his original degree) in a small family firm making cleaning chemicals and stayed there for the rest of his life.

By the age of seven, I had become a holiday laboratory assistant and chemical process worker. It was unpaid except in stale rye buns with thick wedges of elderly salami from the local Polish deli. I learnt to pour concentrated acids and alkalis safely, mouth pipetting and the keeping of careful experimental records. On the factory shop floor, we had a chemical shed, a bottling plant and the offices, three separate and distinct worlds.

As I progressed through A levels, my father changed my career ambitions which had been vaguely focussed on academic science. He announced that I was 'too stupid to be a scientist and so I would have to be a doctor'. This sounds painfully blunt in English but quite straightforward in Slovakian and nicely illustrates the lack of nuance available in more basic Slavonic languages. I was a very bad medical student, sullen, flippant, argumentative, ungracious and lazy. At qualification, the bloody-mindedness turned in on itself and I determined to learn as much as I could in each job and frequent locums in more exotic specialties to 'try something different'. However, the lure of chemistry, the smells, the myriad processes and their unseen dangers remained: very much a first love. Thus, a small ad at the back of the *BMJ* belatedly applied for deposited me in the summer of 1973 as 'assistant works medical officer' at ICI Huddersfield, a sprawling square mile of chemical sheds employing 5000 men (plus three women process workers left over from World War 2).

My senior Medical Officer was Bill Taylor who handed me all the process documentation and all the toxicology books then extant (four) on my first day and told me to make my conclusions when I was ready. On the fourth day, I went back and said, 'There seem to be a lot of gaps'. He said 'Quite right: so off you go and fill them'. My other teachers were Alex Munn and Geoff Shaw from whom I learnt much toxicology and other specialized occupational science. Sadly Geoff Shaw became ill soon after I arrived and I found myself in his place as senior Medical Officer (Toxicology, Temporary, Unpaid). Despite the unplanned entry mechanism, I knew then as I know now that I had found my vocation.

Source: *Occupational Medicine*, Volume 58, Issue 1, January 2008, Page 4, https://doi.org/10.1093/occmed/kqm042. Copyright © The Author 2008.
Reprinted by permission of Oxford University Press on behalf of the Society of Occupational Medicine.

Are you ready for the EU Sharps Directive 2010/32/EU?

Sabine Wicker and Paul Grime

The risks of needlestick injuries are well recognized, but they keep happening. However, new European legislation, Council Directive 2010/32/EU, must be implemented in member states by 11 May 2013. This 'Sharps Directive' aims to achieve '*the safest possible working environment*' by preventing sharps injuries in hospitals and the healthcare sector. To achieve this, a combination of planning, awareness-raising, information, training and monitoring is essential. Continuous reporting systems are needed, including local, national and European-wide systems. Occupational physicians should draw the attention of employers and health care workers to the new legislation and provide practical leadership in implementing it.

The European Biosafety Network, UNISON and the Royal College of Nursing invited international delegates to the 3rd European Biosafety Summit in London on 1 June 2012. The meeting highlighted the importance of the Sharps Directive on the safety of patients and health care workers and provided an opportunity to share best practice on practical steps to prepare for implementation of the Directive (http://europeanbiosafetynetwork.eu). Participants agreed that appropriate strategies can reduce the risk of transmission of bloodborne pathogens such as hepatitis B and C and HIV. But what should these strategies look like? The measures specified in the Directive (training, safer working procedures and the use of safety engineered devices) can prevent most exposures if implemented together and implemented effectively. If any elements are missed though, the impact of the whole programme will be undermined.

Why is the new European legislation important? On 7 June 2012, a nurse working at the University Hospital Frankfurt, Germany, sustained a significant injury from a hollow-bore needle (16 gauge). The source patient had an HIV load of 64,000 copies/ml. The nurse started HIV post-exposure prophylaxis (PEP) within 30 minutes of the incident and was treated as per the hospital's needlestick protocol. On the day of her needlestick injury, the nurse appeared anxious but showed great professional composure. I explained the treatment protocol to her, the laboratory results, the risk of the exposure and the details of the course of HIV PEP. The next morning the nurse called me after spending the 'night on the internet' researching her risk. She hadn't slept and was terrified, saying '*I have never had such a fear!*' I will never forget this sentence; I will never forget her tears.

The emotional impact of needlestick injury should not be underestimated. Several cases of post-traumatic stress disorder (PTSD) have been described after needlestick injuries involving high-risk patients. On average, at least one needlestick injury is reported every day at the University Hospital Frankfurt (519 needlestick injuries were reported between October 2010–April 2012). Almost 90% of source patients are tested for bloodborne pathogens, and more than 20% are found to be infected.

Preventing needlestick injuries is in everybody interest. The Sharps Directive has the potential to reduce the incidence of needlestick injuries. Occupational physicians have a responsibility to make every effort to promote and support its implementation.

Source: *Occupational Medicine*, Volume 63, Issue 2, March 2013, Page 144, https://doi.org/10.1093/occmed/kqs229. Copyright © The Author(s) 2013.

Fifty years ago: 'A poisons information service'

Roy Goulding

In 1961 an official report was published by H.M. Stationery Office on the 'Emergency Treatment of Acute Poisoning in Hospitals'. This was the work of a special committee set up under the Central Health Services Council. After reviewing the statistics and existing arrangements, six specific re-commendations were advanced, and among them was one to the effect that 'An information service on poisoning should be set up with central arrangements for co-ordination'.

In the first place it was considered that the entries should cover medicinal, veterinary, agri-cultural, horticultural and household articles. Then, after discussion with the British Medical Association, it was agreed that industrial items should be added as well. The original reluctance to include this last category arose from the belief that provision was already made in some measure for industrial chemicals, through individual industrial medical officers, the Appointed Factory Doctors of the Ministry of Labour and so on and that, in any event, this was a specialized business to which considerable attention was even then being devoted. Nevertheless, the deci-sion to extend into the industrial field was finally taken, not only, as it were, 'in response to a popular demand' but also because it was understood that many industrial medical officers were of the mind that the advantages to be gained thereby would certainly outweigh any risks of overlapping.

In February 1965, a report was published of the first twelve months' operation of the ser-vice (R. Goulding and R. R. Watkin, 1965). Out of a total of 2100 enquiries handled during this period, only seventy-four were classified as industrial. Scrutiny of these queries individu-ally reveals a diverse assortment, from exposure to sulphur dioxide to splashing with chromic acid, from breathing chlorine to handling caesium chloride, from getting a cyanide test reagent in the mouth to contact with mercury. With one exception there was no distinctive pattern at all and that exception concerned polytetrafluoroethylenes. No less than eight incidents were brought to notice in which workers had inhaled the fumes liberated by heating or burning polytetrafluoroethylene (e.g. 'Fluon', 'Teflon') with the subsequent development of so-called 'polymer fume fever'.

What has emerged from this industrial side, however, is a tendency for more general ques-tions to be asked—the risks of repeated exposure, for example, rather than the management of an acute incident. Inevitably there has been some trespassing into the field of doubtful aetiology. Thus, where a generalized polyneuritis, or unusual encephalitis, has beset a worker the clinicians have asked whether various substances which he has handled might have been contributory to his condition. Strictly speaking, it is not the business of the Service to pronounce on such mat-ters but, under present circumstances, where else can such people be referred? Through some fortunate and largely 'old-boy' contacts with industry and, more especially, its medical advisers, increasing guidance, which one hopes is both reliable and useful, has been advanced in this way.

Nevertheless, looking to the future, it is uncertain how far the Service should really so proceed. And, if it does, what should be its relationship with the Inspectorate of the Ministry of Labour, if embarrassments are to be avoided?

Source: *Occupational Medicine*, Volume 65, Issue 4, June 2015, Page 346, https://doi.org/10.1093/occmed/ kqv031. Copyright © The Author 2015.

Originally from: A poisons information service. *Trans Ass Industr Med Offrs* (1965) 15, 150. Available at: *Occup Med (Lond)* 1965;15:150–151. DOI:10.1093/ occmed/15.1.150.

Tales of Kieran: The occupational physician's odyssey 5—Drivers

J.A. Hunter

'It's that lunatic at the University Occupational Health Department!', my general practitioner friend bellowed whilst we were enjoying a Rioja at Linbridge golf club (purely for our platelets, of course). 'Kieran whatisname. He's started testing liver enzymes on all taxi and bus drivers since he got the council contract. Two of my patients have failed and are looking at losing their jobs. It really isn't on.'

He was clearly upset, but I decided that silence was the best form of diplomacy in the circumstances. The next day, I arranged to have lunch with Kieran at St Arrhenius College to see if I could winkle out anything further. He must have thought I had alcohol on the brain, but none of the bait for a bite and I was beginning to despair over coffee when Kieran said that there was a Lincaster Society of Occupational Medicine meeting on 'Driving and Drugs' next week and why didn't I come along?

It's always good to venture into strange specialities every now and then. Our own grand rounds have become much less interesting eve since old Bob 'Bible' Brooks retired. He used to present the more fabulous and rare cases, and then tell everybody that the miraculous recovery was due to the entire firm praying at the patient's bedside. Besides, a meeting with Kieran present was bound to be interesting.

Fortunately, I met someone I vaguely knew beforehand and was able to sit on the other side of the room from Kieran, where I could get a safe view of the proceedings. I could see him straining on the leash during the presentation, leaping up and down in his seat at certain comments, but somehow restraining himself from shouting out. But after the presentations had finished, he tore into the speaker from the DVLA, calling him a government lackey and demanded to know how he could personally allow thousands of alcoholics on to the roads to drive juggernauts and buses and not even ask them to have a blood test as part of their medical. There then followed a stand-up row between Kieran and a clinical psychologist about the effects of common anti-depressants and reaction times, which ended up with Kieran accusing the psychologist of verbal diarrhoea and having no concept of the real world. There was a general murmur of approval at his last comment. Great stuff!

Afterwards, I went over to congratulate Kieran on a splendid display. He was clearly charged up. 'I need a drink,' he gasped, and we made our way over the road for a half. Kieran was talking so fast and excitedly that I am not sure if he actually drank any of his beer, so I still don't know if alcohol can be implicated in what happened next. Leaving the pub, we climbed into his car. I tried to point it out, but Kieran was still gibbering on about his units and MCVs and gammaGT, and was so excited he obviously wasn't in the state to notice anything else. He started the car and we shot straight across the car park, demolished a section of iron railings and ended up on the college lawn. Whilst alcohol probably wasn't the direct cause, indirectly he fought to take his anti-theft device off his steering wheel. When the man from the DVLA tapped on the window to see if everything was alright, the look on his face when he saw who was behind the wheel said it all.

Source: *Occupational Medicine*, Volume 52, Issue 7, October 2002, Page 417, https://doi.org/10.1093/occmed/52.7.417. Copyright © Society of Occupational Medicine 2002.

Why I became an occupational physician ...

Hans Engel

In 1935 I had the good fortune to be able to leave Nazi Germany and study medicine at the only British medical school, in Edinburgh, which accepted refugees. Just before I was due to qualify, I was interned for 9 months in Canada due to a mix-up between POWs, 'enemy' and 'friendly' aliens.

After returning to Scotland and qualifying, my German name impeded me getting a job, but after 50 unsuccessful applications I got started as a casualty officer in Rotherham, at £50 for 6 months. There I had plenty of 'industrial' experience such as amputated fingers at wire works and other factories, which did not practise much 'health and safety' at the time.

After serving for 4 years in the British Army in France, Belgium, Holland and a very defeated Germany, the state subsidized vocational study for veterans. I took several postgraduate courses but then failed in the membership exams three times! So I could not become an internist, which was my first choice of career. I had met Ronald Lane when I was just a houseman in Salford, but he did not at that time have much influence on my career. But then Nigel Douglas persuaded me to take the Diploma in Industrial Health in Edinburgh, my alma mater, which in those days usefully comprised the Certificate of Public Health. Armed with my 'DIH' I soon settled in my new discipline and was lucky to obtain a very versatile job in Slough and subsequently at Ford Motors.

Fifty years ago 'Industrial Medicine' really was a Cinderella among medical specialities, and doctors often entered it 'faute de mieux' when they could not obtain a specialist or hospital appointment.

Our exemplars, like Thackrah, Lane and Donald Hunter, specialized mostly in industrial or occupational diseases. Nowadays, occupational medicine deals with many subspecialities, so that we have aviation medicine, sports medicine, armed forces, environmental medicine, rehabilitation and toxicology, which in my early days used to be all part of 'Industrial Medicine'.

I have always had interests in a wide variety of fields, covered by internal medicine, general practice and later by occupational medicine, which were also practised at Fords, where I spent the next 27 years. There I had the opportunity to run a contact dermatitis clinic and publish papers on such diverse subjects as haematology, neurology, emergency medicine, toxicology and accident proneness.

So I have no regrets that I chose 'Industrial Medicine', which, even though at the time second best, has since turned out, by serendipity, to have been the ideal choice for me.

Source: *Occupational Medicine*, Volume 58, Issue 2, March 2008, Page 151, https://doi.org/10.1093/occmed/kqm084. Copyright © The Author 2008.

The ex-service men's maternity ward

John D. Meyer

This picture (Figure 88.1) was taken in about 1969 whilst cycling through the Sangli District in southern Maharashtra state, India. I am unsure if the building stands any longer. The maternity ward was evidently built as an adjunct to the Sangli Civil Hospital for the benefit of veterans' families, and accompanied a rest-home and hostel serving the same group [1]. Though clearly, and unironically, constructed 'to care for him who shall have borne the battle and for his widow and his orphan', in the words of Lincoln's Second Inaugural Address [2], 40 years on we may see its purpose very differently. Women soldiers serve in India in similar positions as in the USA, UK and most other countries, though not without familiar debate as to their role in combat. Women's health and maternity care therefore becomes a benefit of their own service, rather than a family perquisite of the male soldier's commission.

My own odd-ball thoughts on the picture, though, stem from my work in the epidemiology of occupational hazards in pregnancy. Evidence has slowly built that work tasks and exposures vary by gender, even within the ostensibly same job title [3]. Here is the golden opportunity to have a counterfactual population to study and contrast with my own subjects, namely men who have become pregnant. Just imagine the research questions that might be answered therein.

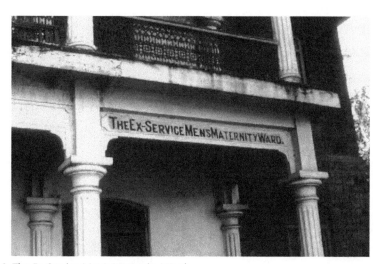

Figure 88.1 The Ex-Service Men's Maternity Ward
Reproduced with permission from Meyer J. D. (2013). The ex-service men's maternity ward. *Occup Med (Lond)*. **63**(2):140, https://doi.org/10.1093/occmed/kqs221

References

1. **Sangli District**. *Maharashtra State Gazetteers*. Bombay: Directorate of Government Printing, Stationery and Publications, 1969. http://cultural.maharashtra.gov.in/ english/gazetteer/SANGLI/gen_admin_collector.html 10 October 2012, date last accessed).

2. **Lincoln A.** *Second Inaugural Address*. Washington DC. Library of Congress, 1865. http://www.loc.gov/rr/ program/bib/ourdocs/Lincoln2nd.html (11 December 2012, date last accessed).

3. **Messing K, Silverstein BA.** Gender and occupational health. *Scand J Work Environ Health* 2009;35:81–83.

Source: *Occupational Medicine*, Volume 63, Issue 2, March 2013, Page 140, https://doi.org/10.1093/occmed/kqs221. Copyright © The Author 2013.

Medicine is my lawful wife, and literature is my mistress

Nerys Williams

Our subject has been described both as one of the world's five greatest dramatists and as one of the world's five greatest short story writers [1]. In his short life, he produced brilliant plays and stories, yet he spent most of his adult years as a practising physician.

Born in 1860 in the Soviet Union, he was initially educated at a school for Greek boys [2] but the family descended into poverty when his father was declared bankrupt in 1876. He paid for his own education through a succession of jobs including private tutoring, catching birds and selling short stories. In 1884, he qualified in medicine from Moscow University and worked in hospitals. He really wanted to become a lecturer at the medical school and so undertook a medico-social study of a penal colony to gain his doctorate. Over a 3-month period, he interviewed 6000 people reporting on their social conditions. What he found appalled him. The inhabitants lived in conditions of poor sanitation and very low standards of public health. There were epidemics of diphtheria and typhoid and cases of pneumonia, marasmus and gastrointestinal disorders. He recognized that the poor social conditions produced ill-health and stated publicly that the role of the physician was not to treat patients but to eliminate the adverse social conditions that reduced resistance to disease. He concluded that charity and subscription were not the answer but that government had a duty to finance human treatment for the less fortunate convicts.

The university ultimately rejected his thesis and our subject gave up academic medicine although he published his thesis privately [3]. In 1892, he bought a small country estate, built three schools and donated his medical services for the good of the peasants despite experiencing his own ill-health. His work as a doctor both enriched his writing but left him little time to write as much as he wished.

In the beginning, his literary output was not very successful. In 1896, he renounced the theatre after the disastrous reception of one of his most famous plays only for it to receive acclaim just two years later, despite challenging both the actors and the audience. At first, he wrote stories for the money but he became more artistic and innovative, insisting that the role of an artist was to ask questions and not to answer them [4].

In March 1897, he suffered a haemorrhage of the lungs from tuberculosis, undoubtedly contracted from the penal colony. He moved to Yalta and continued to write but by May 1904 he was terminally ill. His death was as dramatic as some of his plays—he sat up, his doctor gave him an injection of camphor, he drank a glass of champagne, then lay on his left side and quietly, like a child sleeping, he passed away. Anton Chekhov did nothing, except with style.

References

1. **Galton DJ.** Anton Chekhov's MD thesis. *QJM* 1981;**11**:43–47.
2. Wikipedia. Anton Chekhov. www.wikipedia.org/wiki/Anton_Chekhov (14 March 2009, date last accessed).

3. **Checkhov AP.** *The Island: A Journey to Sakhalin.* New York: Washington Square Press, 1975.

4. **Bartlett R, Phillips A.** (translators). *Chekhov: A Life in Letters.* London: Penguin Books, 2004.

Source: *Occupational Medicine*, Volume 59, Issue 6, September 2009, Page 368, https://doi.org/10.1093/occmed/kqp052. Copyright © The Author 2009.

Those two impostors

Anthony Seaton

Two dates, 5 August and 13 October 2010, defined the 69 days between the disaster of the roof collapse in the San Jose copper mine in Chile and the triumph of the rescue of the 33 trapped miners. Watching the men coming, one by one, to the surface to be greeted by their families after an ordeal unimaginable to most of us, Kipling's words kept coming back to me: 'If you can meet with Triumph and Disaster, and treat those two impostors just the same ...'. The men, young and old met the disaster of near certainty of a slow death with remarkable equanimity, aided by their religious faith and inspired leadership. The rescue from entombment half a mile underground was a triumph of engineering and of disaster management by the Chilean authorities. Now the men have to face the problems of the triumph.

Miners are hardy, self-reliant folk, following their fathers into the pit, as few other employment opportunities exist in their community. These communities conceal a similar range of talent and intelligence to be found in any better educated group, including those who sit in Parliament, as witness their brass bands, choirs, rugby and political debates. I once met a Staffordshire miner who had taught himself Latin and Greek in order to read the Classics in the original. But they differ from the rest of us in having to face risk of death every day they go to work. Before nation-alization, mine explosions and fires were commonplace in the UK, often killing hundreds of men. Even the communities share in hazard; in 1966, the collapse of a tip at Aberfan killed 144 people, including 116 school children. Poor nutrition, relative poverty, air pollution and sometimes poor medical services lead to an unhealthy population, at the mercy of economic forces outwith their control.

The triumph of the rescue in Copiapó conceals a sadder story, of failure to control risk. Two of the men were found to have silicosis—presumably, no health surveillance had been carried out. The men were being paid danger money in a mine notoriously liable to rock falls. Those 33 men rescued are matched each year by an average of 33 deaths in the Chilean copper mines, increasing as previously unsafe private mines reopen because of rising copper prices.

It is well to remember to whom we owe our prosperity, at a time when people are being put out of work. They are not those who speculate in money, but those who produce the necessities of modern life. Among these are the miners of Chile who produce one-third of the world's copper, essential to communications, to construction and even to brass bands. They will never drink champagne in their yachts. Any day, an accident could deprive them of their lives or their liveli-hood. And we are the consumers for whom they run these risks. We rely on them, in good times and bad. Health and safety is not the joke some in the media take it to be.

Source: *Occupational Medicine*, Volume 61, Issue 1, January 2011, Page 70, https://doi.org/10.1093/occmed/kqq179. Copyright © The Author 2010.

Why I became an occupational physician …

Athol Hepburn

I have read with great interest the accounts given by various occupational physicians, on their reasons for entering occupational medicine. Perhaps my own career, which involved a more positive choice than serendipity, will add to the pot pourri.

In the 1950s, I applied for a short service commission in the Royal Navy in order to enter my preferred choice of service. After some 2 years at sea, including the Gulf and East Indies, I moved to the Fleet Air Arm, specializing in aviation medicine. On leaving the regular navy, I transferred to the London Division of the Royal Naval Reserve, where I served for a further 24 years.

In 1960, I invested in a year's study at the London School of Hygiene and Tropical Medicine, where I was fortunate to be taught by Richard Schilling and Austin Bradford Hill. This enabled me to be appointed to the British Overseas Airway Corporation. My main job there was looking after flying staff. I was for many years an authorized medical examiner, although I was seconded for a short period as medical adviser to the emerging Nigeria Airways in Lagos.

I became senior medical officer at Royal Aircraft Establishment Farnborough, the home of British aviation. Then in 1972, following political changes in the Heath Administration, I was appointed Director of Civilian Medical Services in the Procurement Executive of the Ministry of Defence, a post I held for some 14 years. This involved running one of the largest multidisciplinary occupational health services in the UK and arguably the most diverse, covering some 40 sites. I was fortunate in having a talented team of occupational physicians, occupational health nurses and occupational hygienists.

I chaired the Ministry of Defence Occupational Health Committee for 11 years. Another interest was as Chairman of the Royal Navy's Underwater Personnel Research Committee, whose work on deep saturation diving was conducted at the Royal Naval Physiological Laboratory.

My work also led to my membership for some 10 years of the Anglo-French Concorde Aeromedical Subcommittee. These were exciting years, when one felt, albeit in a small way, part of the cutting edge of aerospace technology.

At sixty, I was able to work part time at the Atomic Weapons Establishment in Aldermaston, part of my old bailiwick, for doctors I had appointed and helped to train. This is sometimes called role reversal and was for me salutary.

The seeds of my interest in Occupational Medicine were sown at Aberdeen University and flourished in the armed services. My positive choice enabled me to work with, and for, some of the best scientific and engineering talents in the UK and offered a variety of challenges denied to many.

Source: *Occupational Medicine*, Volume 58, Issue 3, May 2008, Page 154, https://doi.org/10.1093/occmed/kqn016. Copyright © The Author 2008.

An elusive occupational toxin

Hans Engel

While I was working at Ford Motor Co we used to carry out routine annual blood counts, lead levels, chest x-rays and urinalysis on all paint sprayers. In 1977 my technician alerted me to the presence of an unusual number of operators showing much reduced neutrophils. The most likely cause to an occupational physician would be benzene. So I persuaded our chemists to work through the weekend analysing all 53 paints, thinners and solvents available in the paintshop. But no benzene was discovered. Then a nurse remarked to me that curiously some of the workmen had French names. It emerged that these all came from the Antilles in the West Indies, and I wondered whether this could be a genetic abnormality. Searching the literature I found that neutropenia had only been mentioned among Africans and to a very minor degree in African-Americans, but not in other countries. We reassured our workers that they were not being poisoned, and I published a short article in the *Journal of the Royal Society of Medicine* to alert other occupational physicians.

Soon afterwards a paediatrician in Bristol wrote to me to say he had seen this in adults with rheumatoid arthritis and children with Felty's syndrome. He had found that an intravenous bolus of cortisone would rectify the condition. I tried this on myself and felt no ill effects, so I offered this procedure to 20 of the paintsprayers involved. Incredibly, they all consented and were given 100mg of hydrocortisone. Four hours later their neutrophils had all been raised to normal.

I since understand that in many Africans some neutrophils tend to adhere to the blood vessel wall in what is called 'laking'.

When I think back 35 years later it still amazes me that everybody consented without demur or a randomized control trial. Today I shudder to think how the General Medical Council or trade union would castigate this procedure. It was disappointing that there were no occupational causes, but it quickly reassured the workers. A sobering thought is that this had all been anticipated in George Bernard Shaw's *The Doctor's Dilemma*, produced in 1906, where Sir Ralph Bloomfield Bonington famously states 'There is at bottom only one genuinely *scientific* treatment for all diseases, and that is to stimulate the phagocytes.'

Nothing new under the sun?

Source: *Occupational Medicine,* Volume 63, Issue 3, April 2013, Page 182, https://doi.org/10.1093/occmed/kqt004. Copyright © The Author 2013.

Fifty years ago: 'The Proposed New Constitution'

Anon

Some years ago the Council of the Association set up a Working Party (in what way does a Working Party differ from a Committee?) to consider the Constitution of the Association and to make recommendations. The Working Party is now nearing the end of its work and before long the members of the Association will be asked to consider the new constitution it has recommended.

We need a new constitution because our Association has grown too big for the old one, and because occupational medicine has increased greatly in importance, or at least in recognition, over the last thirty or so years. So the new constitution is more formal and more precise; it is longer, duller and by no means light reading—but after all it is not intended to be read as light entertainment.

At present the Association is run by the Council— only the Council can take official decisions, answer official questions, consider bright ideas about the Association and about occupational medicine generally. And the Council is too big: for some years it has been plain that it must be relieved of most of the minor decisions, otherwise nothing will get done. So the officers, informally and unofficially, have been acting as a kind of executive committee. In fact, the need for a properly constituted Executive Committee has been demonstrated and the obvious thing to do is to set one up. But the Executive Committee will be concerned with the day to day affairs of the Association: we need some other working committees or panels to be responsible for particular parts of the Association's work. The Working Party says 'These Panels should be active in their own right, they should be prepared to originate action within their own fields: not merely to deliberate on matters referred to them.

Another change recommended is the reduction of the President's term of office from two years to one year. The job has become too heavy a burden to ask a man to carry for two years. Moreover, the term of two years prevents many suitable people from ever becoming President.

But these changes and others of minor details are, in one way, less important than the proposed change of title. If this new Executive Committee turns out in practice to be wrongly constituted, it can easily be put right: the Association cannot change its title every few years. So the title chosen now will have to remain for a very long time. It is suggested that the 'medical officer' has now the wrong implications, that 'occupational medicine' is more accurate than 'industrial medicine' and that 'Society' is better than 'Association'. This leads to 'Society of Occupational Medicine'. It is a good ringing mouthful: if the members accept the new constitution and with it the new title that will be at least a step towards better occupational medicine in this country. Not, however, a very long step as yet.

Source: *Occupational Medicine*, Volume 65, Issue 4, June 2015, Page 345, https://doi.org/10.1093/occmed/kqv030. Copyright © The Author 2015.

Originally from: The Proposed New Constitution. *Occup Med (Lond)* 1965;15:1. DOI:10.1093/occmed/15.1.1.

Armadillo

John Hobson

A firmly established tradition of the American Occupational Health Conference is the 'Britpack' dinner; the Society of Occupational Medicine hosts a return fixture at the Annual Scientific Meeting. We were in Orlando debating the finer points of the scientific programme when talk turned to golf. Previously the 14th hole on the conference hotel course had boasted an argumentative alligator who was eventually relocated to Gatorland where he lives to this day. Gatorland is worth a visit if only for the bird life and the boardwalk through virgin everglade rather than the bizarre sight of a man wrestling a huge reptile. But my American co-diner Warner said that an even stranger golf hazard was the armadillo. He had hit one once and not only did the ball ping off the hard leathery shell never to be seen again but the animal flew four feet into the air. This is something they do when startled often to impressive and destructive effect under motor vehicles. However Warner continued, and to ensure we could all claim our CPD points with a clear conscience, the armadillo is the cause of an occupational disease. A 2011 study in the *New England Journal of Medicine* confirmed that armadillos can transmit *Mycobacterium leprae* to humans. They are the only animals known to carry leprosy due to their low body temperature which provides a good environment for the bacteria and in humans M. *leprae* prefers cooler areas, such as nostrils, fingers and toes. The armadillo first became a host for leprosy following introduction of the bacteria to South America by European settlers. Leprosy, or Hansen's disease, named after the Norwegian physician Gerhard Armauer Hansen, is a granulomatous disease of the peripheral nerves and mucosa of the upper respiratory tract; skin lesions are the primary external sign. In the USA, there are 250 cases of leprosy reported each year of which a third are attributable to armadillos. The zoonosis can be contracted as a result of shooting them, eating infected meat or through the shell which is made into a musical instrument by indigenous South Americans and sought after in the USA as a souvenir. The occupational link is in those who handle them through farming or research work. Mycobacterium leprae is extremely hard to grow and for that reason the armadillo is used in research laboratories although laboratory workers are adequately protected if they have had the BCG vaccination. Diagnosis in the USA is often delayed because health-care providers are unaware of leprosy and its symptoms. Early diagnosis and treatment prevents nerve involvement and the disability it causes. Left untreated, leprosy can be progressive, causing permanent damage to the skin, nerves, limbs and eyes. Worldwide, 2–3 million people are estimated to be permanently disabled because of leprosy. Even though global incidence is now falling, in 2000, the World Health Organization (WHO) listed 91 countries in which Hansen's disease was endemic with India, Burma and Nepal containing 70% of cases. The things you learn at conferences.

Source: *Occupational Medicine*, Volume 64, Issue 3, April 2014, Page 222, https://doi.org/10.1093/occmed/kqu013. Copyright © The Author 2014.

Why I became an occupational physician …

Tim Carter

In short: because I could not arrange a winter elective in Malta and went to ICI at Runcorn instead!

When my aims of an elective in the sun fell through, I had just been on a visit to a cattle cake mill in East London—UCH's gesture towards occupational medicine—and been fascinated with a study in progress there to see if workers who handled tetracyclines, then a permitted feed additive, had resistant organisms in their noses and throats.

At school I had been interested in the processes of the chemical industry, largely from a text-book written by T. M. Lowry, later to become my 'grandfather in law'. From school I had also visited a hellish gasworks, now under the millennium dome, and M and Bs smelly sulphapyridine production plant in Dagenham. So when my elective was 2 weeks away, I thought of the chemical industry and wrote to Lloyd Potter, Chief Medical Officer, of ICI. I had a rather awesome visit to a large office in their Millbank HQ and a week later was with David Duffield, the plant Medical Officer of ICI Castner Kellner who works at Runcorn. This was the start of a month when I visited everything from Cheshire salt mines to laboratories studying the strange toxicology of paraquat, then a new herbicide. I was brilliantly looked after and educated. What drew me back to occupational medicine later was the wide range of clever and analytical people, working together in a climate where the doctor was valued for their skills but could not luxuriate in what, as a medical student, looked like the professional arrogance of most clinical consultants. Lloyd Potter gave me some advice that was easy to follow. 'Spend a few years getting general experience anywhere in the world and then do the DIH'. I happily went round the world for 3 years and then saw the advert for the London School of Hygiene MSc course, returned to the UK and got stuck in.

My early years in the trade were spent working first for a Swann (Peter at Esso, but Ward Gardner at Fawley was my role model and mentor there), then a Duck (Bertie at BP Sunbury) and a Heron (Peter a chemical engineer at BP chemicals). At BP Chemicals, I caught up with most of the doctors I had met at ICI nearly a decade earlier as BP Chemicals and ICI came to grips with the management of the angiosarcoma risks from vinyl chloride. Were we protecting workers, the chemical industry or both? I am still not sure but it was a great team with worldwide connections.

Then, with Ken Duncan's encouragement, to Health & Safety Executive as their medical director. Lots of satisfaction and not many regrets, but a recognition that in occupational health 'to everything there is a season'. You have to grab the opportunity to act in the short periods when, as was the case with vinyl chloride risks, everyone is crying out for expertise to deal with a pressing problem.

Source: *Occupational Medicine*, Volume 58, Issue 3, May 2008, Page 224, https://doi.org/10.1093/occmed/kqm056. Copyright © The Author 2008.

Reprinted by permission of Oxford University Press on behalf of the Society of Occupational Medicine.

Learning from the Vikings: Hávamál and occupational rehabilitation

Desmond O'Neill

Although the pioneering work of Bernardo Ramazzini is often cited as the origin of occupational health, an awareness of some aspects of occupational illness dates back to classical times [1]. Hippocrates described lead poisoning, and Pliny was aware of the poisonous nature of sulphur, mercury and lead.

Our first historical insight into a different aspect of occupational health arises from a surprising source, one of the first of the Viking sagas. Viking culture suffers unfairly from images of savage warriors with horned helmets intent on rape and pillage wherever their beautiful ships bore them. One might imagine that their addition to the lore of medicine would be more likely to arise in emergency medicine and trauma orthopaedics.

Yet as visitors to Dublin and York will know, the Vikings led remarkably sophisticated lives within a highly organized and structured culture. From one of their most ancient of Norse poetic sagas, *Hávamál* [2], we find a wisdom that points to one of the key aspects of occupational health, how to overcome the hurdle of diagnosis as catastrophe and occupational rehabilitation to the workplace. This extended and often very droll poem was handed down in oral tradition, purportedly from the Norse god Odin—what better authority could we ask for?—and is a sequence of pithy advice and wise counsels. In addition to guidance on the perils of drunkenness, visitors out-staying their welcome and the virtues of silence, a number of stanzas deal with illness.

After a nod to preventive medicine—'These things are thought the best:/....,/Good health with the gift to keep it,/And a life that avoids vice'—we are reassured by the importance of family support and what remains in illness: 'Not all sick men are utterly wretched:/Some are blessed with sons,/Some with friends,/some with riches,/Some with worthy works'. The contrast with the alternative is always present: 'It is always better to be alive,/The living can keep a cow./Fire, I saw, warming a wealthy man,/With a cold corpse at his door'.

But the true spark lies in the promotion of adaptation of acquired disability to certain types of occupation: 'The halt can manage a horse,/the handless a flock,/The deaf be a doughty fighter'. These wonderful images should reassure us that the mission of occupational medicine builds on a tradition that is considerably older than we may have imagined.

And although we would never be so blunt in practice, the steely truth of the stanza's final line—'/ To be blind is better than to burn on a pyre/There is nothing the dead can do'—is an unspoken motivation that we all too rarely articulate.

References

1. **Abrams HK.** A short history of occupational health. *J Public Health Policy* 2001;**22**:34–80.
2. Anonymous. Hávamál circa 800–900AD.

Source: *Occupational Medicine*, Volume 63, Issue 3, April 2013, Page 230, https://doi.org/10.1093/occmed/kqs230. Copyright © The Author 2013.

Early thoughts on g

Mike Gibson

Towards the end of the First World War, the average life expectancy of a pilot at the Western Front was around 17 days [1]. There was concern that medical unfitness was contributing to the attrition rate. A conference to discuss the issues was held on 27th February 1917, chaired by Fleet Surgeon R. C. Munday, RN, soon to be appointed the first head of the RAF Medical Service. The conference concentrated on the symptoms of high flying, acclimatization and the use of oxygen equipment as well as the development of medical standards for pilots. The studies that followed led to the publication of *The Medical Problems of Flying* after the war, which focused on hypoxia and the psychological aspects of aviation but did not address protection against gravitational forces (g) applied in the head to foot direction (gz). Although Head [2] described greying out, blacking out and even possible loss of consciousness during aerobatic manoeuvres, he reported considerable variation between pilots, and the only suggestion made was the problems could be overcome by adaptation and experience.

However, in discussion following a meeting of the Medical Society of London in early 1918 [3], Munday drew attention to the importance of the posture of the aviator during a steep spiral. He stated that in the usual upright position, 'the centrifugal action must seriously affect the cerebral blood pressure'. He went on to suggest that if the pilot 'leant back as far as possible centrifugal action on the brain' would be 'almost nil'. Development of g protection in the UK was not really considered until the 1930s. From then on, research concentrated successively on muscle tensing, abdominal belts, raising the rudder pedals, the development of air- and fluid-filled anti-g suits and, for a time, prone position aircraft. Munday's practical comments appear to have been the first published advice on gz protection. However, possibly because he only lasted 6 months in his role as head of the new RAF Medical Service, the suggestion proved to be a cul de sac in the road to gz protection until, independently, the Americans designed the ACES II ejection seat for the F-16 with a seat back angle of 30° in the 1970s. How did Munday, a career Naval doctor with no experience of flying, know about gz? His son, R. B. Munday, flew Sopwith Camels in the Royal Naval Air Service and was a recognized 'ace', holding the Distinguished Service Cross. This gives a different slant to the adage that it is not what you know but who you know that counts.

References

1. **Barker R.** *The Royal Flying Corps in World War I.* London: Robinson, 2002; **223**, 278.
2. **Head H.** The sense of stability and balance in the air. In: *The Medical Problems of Flying.* London: MedicalResearch Council, 1920; 214–256.
3. **Anderson HG.** Aviation and medicine and the selection of candidates for the air force. *Lancet* 1918;i:407.

Source: *Occupational Medicine*, Volume 63, Issue 3, April 2015, Page 189, https://doi.org/10.1093/occmed/kqu089. Copyright © The Author 2015.

Reprinted by permission of Oxford University Press on behalf of the Society of Occupational Medicine.

Employers—aren't they all the same?

John Challenor

Listening to employees day after day, one might be forgiven for believing that all employers are tarred with the same brush. Here is a story about two employees who reminded me of how organizations can and do treat their workers differently.

Explaining to the first patient that their convalescence ought to be coming to an end, I had initiated an exploration of some avenues for a phased return to work. But why was this employee so reluctant to return to labour for the organization that had supported her sickness absence and would provide the means to put food on the table and allow ample paid annual leave for all manner of exotic holidays? What had spawned such disenchantment and antipathy? Had the milk of human kindness boiled over or just evaporated? It turned out that these metaphors were uncomfortably close to the truth. There had been cutbacks, spending constraints, rising costs and targets. Staff who had left had not been replaced. The directorate administrator had decreed that milk would no longer be provided for staff during tea or coffee breaks. To add some fibre to the overworked metaphor, it was simply the last straw when staff had to create a milk rota requiring the purchase and carriage of several litres of milk. My patient explained, 'They want more and more and offer less and less in return. I don't feel up to going back just yet'.

A similar situation was illustrated by 'Can He Fix It?' Sir Gerry Robinson when the night shift staff in a nursing home had been reprimanded for having a slice of toast with their 3.0 a.m. break. Bitter disenchantment was the result. 'We're not even worth a slice of toast!'

Soon after, another employee came to see me. This time a worker who wanted to return to work before his convalescence period ended. 'I feel quite well and really need to get back. We're already a team member down due to maternity leave and I know my colleagues are putting in extra hours. It's not right that I should be sitting at home when I could be sitting at work and sharing the load.'

So what made these two similar workers so different? The employer of the second patient overtly valued each employee. Free breakfast was provided before each morning shift. Free lunch was provided during the day shift and free supper during the late shift or for those working overtime. Free beverages and fruit were available always.

The second employee reminded me of the wise words of another Knight of the Realm, Sir John Harvey-Jones, who said that you get the best out of people when you work with them. Just the other day, I discovered that the second patient worked for an employer that had been in the Sunday Times '100 Best Small Companies to Work For' list for three years in a row. Now why was not I surprised by that?

Source: *Occupational Medicine*, Volume 60, Issue 6, September 2010, Page 420, https://doi.org/10.1093/occmed/kqq059. Copyright © The Author 2010.

Why I became an occupational physician ...

Roy Archibald

I had been called up in the later stages of the Second World War having qualified at Glasgow, where my father had qualified before me, and came home from the Middle East in April 1947. Doctors were flooding out of the three services and looking apprehensively at this new creature, the National Health Service (NHS), which Nye Bevan had taken through parliament. My ship home was an old Castle Line tub, the 'Dunnotar Castle', and on it I decided that (i) I liked clinical medicine, (ii) I believed in prevention and (iii) the Army had given me a taste for administration. I decided that I could find all three in the comparatively new and largely unrecognized specialty of industrial medicine.

I went back to my alma mater and was more than fortunate to find a 1-year course in industrial medicine in the Department of Social Medicine headed by Prof. Tom Ferguson. The course was run by the charismatic Andrew Meiklejohn and in June 1948 I was awarded the DIH by the Faculty of Physicians and Surgeons of Glasgow.

I immediately obtained a post with the alkali division of ICI, then the bellwether of post-war UK industry. We were the wealthiest division, making invaluable US dollars shipping alkali to the eastern seaboard of the States cheaper than they could rail-freight it from the west. I was recruited at the princely salary of £1000 per annum when the British Medical Association recommended figure was £850. I was the junior of three doctors (all Scots) in the division based at Northwich in Cheshire. There were also three dentists (with one of whom I am still in touch) and we were all ICI employees. But advancement in ICI in those days was slow. Movement between divisions was rare and 'dead men's shoes' was the common means of promotion, so after 4.5 years I decided it was time to move on.

After a false start I moved to the National Coal Board in Yorkshire, the roughest, toughest and largest of the eight divisions of the industry. That was in 1953 and there I stayed, moving first to County Durham and then to headquarters in London until retiring at almost 65 in 1985. I worked for the NHS locally until the age of 70 years and then did consultant work until I was 80 years. Now in New Zealand I can look back on a happy career which I much enjoyed and which fully satisfied my desire for clinical medicine, prevention and administration.

Source: *Occupational Medicine*, Volume 58, Issue 4, June 2008, Page 235, https://doi.org/10.1093/occmed/kqm081. Copyright © The Author 2008.
Reprinted by permission of Oxford University Press on behalf of the Society of Occupational Medicine.

The rewards of rural training in the Scottish Highlands

Syed Nasir

When I accepted a four-year training post in NHS Highland I was uncertain about the quality of occupational health (OH) training I would receive in the most remote and mountainous parts of Scotland. However, I had not foreseen the numerous benefits of working in this region.

The NHS Highland OH department is a major OH provider in the area, despite its relatively small size compared with other NHS departments nationally. This helped it win a large range of contracts not usually encountered by many trainees working predominantly with one large public or private sector organization. In contrast, I dealt with a swathe of public sector contracts (NHS, the frontline bluelight services, central/local government and higher education); private sector organizations (from small- and medium-sized enterprises to multinationals) as well as subcontracted work from numerous national OH organizations.

The greatest challenge was covering an area the size of Belgium, taking seven hours to drive from the southernmost clinic in Campbelltown to the northernmost one in Wick. However, it was a privilege to be paid to travel to work in hired cars and ferries across the Scottish West Coast and mountain ranges.

The most enjoyable role was to support the Highland and Island Fire & Rescue Service across this huge area in dealing with the largest retained firefighter workforce in the UK. The logistical acrobatics required to service this contract were extremely interesting, particularly in the numerous remote islands in the Western and Northern Isles. An added dimension was that OH issues were often scrutinized in the local press. One particularly rewarding case was the successful rehabilitation to full duties of possibly the only known retained firefighter in the world with a prosthetic hand.

Potential conflicts of interests commonly occur in rural settings, posing ethical dilemmas such as the referring manager also being a relative or general practitioner of the employee. It can be challenging to maintain confidentiality as employees frequently have multiple roles in related organizations such as a council worker who is a retained firefighter. It is often an advantage being regarded as an 'independent' outsider in more remote areas.

In terms of my MFOM/MSc research, one advantage of this remote location was the ease of access to a relatively research-naïve population and obtaining a third of the local NHS endowment research funding. The Scottish training programme ensured I was not isolated from other Scottish trainees whilst viewing a wide range of interesting workplaces.

Despite its remote location, the department was forward-thinking in developing a four-tiered psychological service for the NHS and researching occupational teledermatology across rural locations.

It was a steep learning curve dealing with sensitive cases and outbreaks of reported occupational symptoms, many of which were scrutinized in the national mainstream and medical media.

All in all, it was an eye-opening experience for all the right reasons. Most of all, my trainers, Dr Steve Ryder and Dr Mark Hilditch, and the team made my time extremely enjoyable.

Source: *Occupational Medicine*, Volume 63, Issue 7, October 2013, Page 478, https://doi.org/10.1093/occmed/kqt096. Copyright © The Author 2013.

Fifty years ago: 'Genesis of a new society'

Anon

It was with some surprise that we recently found ourselves taken to task—privately, and in a most gentle and courteous fashion—for our last leading article. The tone of this was clearly favourable to the proposed new constitution, and our critic felt that we should have withheld editorial judgment until the matter had been voted upon; it was also suggested that we went too far in anticipating an affirmative decision. We are unrepentant. An explicit editorial bias on any important issue is surely to be preferred to one which is subtly concealed, and still more to an attempt to avoid polemics altogether which, in the words of a recent Private Member's motion in Parliament, may result in 'non-controversial pap'. Our views on such subjects as the war in Vietnam may well be influenced by the editorial attitude of our daily newspaper, because we rely on it for facts as well as opinions; it is improbable that we should accord equal weight to the view that health services at work were an instrument of capitalist exploitation, or a mere fringe benefit of affluent industries, because such statements would run counter to our personal experience.

Hence it can hardly be said either that the majority which voted for the new constitution at the March Special General Meeting of the Association was improperly influenced by our support, or that the minority which opposed the changes—perhaps not all for the same reasons—was hamstrung because of it. We respect the motives of this minority, as well as the force of some of their criticisms; but since no constitution in a dynamic body will ever be perfect, we must expect motions to amend parts of it from time to time, and these will no doubt be forthcoming from the critics—to whom also the correspondence columns of this journal are open.

And so from next October we are to become the Society of Occupational Medicine, a title which for a while will have a strange sound. Two of the Panels (Advisory and Educational) have already started their work, and produced important memoranda which would in the past either have been drawn up by the officers or necessitated the setting up of *ad hoc* sub-committees. 'Undoubtedly an increasing number of similar tasks will come their way, and they have advisedly and deliberately been given powers to initiate study of policy problems without having to await formal instructions.

For this and many other provisions designed to enhance the influence of the Society on the contemporary national scene, we must pay tribute to the vision, draughtsmanship and industry of Dr Fisher and his colleagues, who have met in committee no fewer than twenty-six times to produce the constitution which has 'now been approved'.

All in all this is an exciting and stimulating period in which to be alive; and it is good that we have equipped ourselves more adequately to meet its challenge.

Source: *Occupational Medicine*, Volume 65, Issue 5, July 2015, Page 390, https://doi.org/10.1093/occmed/kqv032. Copyright © The Author 2015.

Originally from: *Occup Med (Lond)* 1965;15:41. DOI: 10.1093/occmed/15.1.41.

The mill reek in 1754

Anthony Seaton

To historians and philosophers, Edinburgh is perhaps best known for being the centre of the Scottish Enlightenment. To its inhabitants, until recently, it was known as 'Auld Reekie', acknowledging its smoky atmosphere. Those of us who take an occupational history have heard the Scots words 'stour', for dust and 'reek', for smoke. Indeed, a friendly wish in Scots is 'Lang may your pipe reek'. Well, we know a lot about stour and reek now, and it is certainly best to avoid living or working in an atmosphere of either. I have spent much of my career examining their effects on health, but one type of reek I have seen little of was that from lead refining. Ramazzini drew attention to lead poisoning in De Morbis Artificum Diatriba of 1714 and was quoted on the subject in Pott's 1775 account of scrotal cancer in chimney sweeps, but I doubt that lead poisoning was well known in Britain in that era.

The Enlightenment led to a number of societies in Edinburgh. The Philosophical Society, founded in 1738, became the Royal Society of Edinburgh in 1783. In 1754, it published three volumes of Essays and Observations, edited by Alexander Munro primus and David Hume. These rare books contain, *inter alia*, the first chemical description of a gas, carbon dioxide, by Joseph Black, observations on the moons of Jupiter and an account of how a patient cured himself of secondary syphilis by taking double the recommended dose of mercury. Occupational medicine was not forgotten. James Wilson, surgeon, wrote:

> *'I send what I have observed concerning the disease which the people at Leadhills call the mill-reek, and which all the inhabitants there are subject to; but it mostly seizes, and violently affects the men whose daily business it is to melt down the lead. The melting houses, where this is done are called mills; because the bellows there are worked by water-mills.'*

He then describes abdominal pain, clammy skin, colic, a sweet taste, constipation, loss of appetite, giddiness, headache, delirium and death. He points out:

> *'Thereek or smoak rising from the melting lead is believed to be the cause of this disease; because the melters who are most exposed to the smoak which comes out often full in their faces, are most subject to this disease, the mill-reek. The people here say they have seen birds, in a calm moist day, attempting to fly thro' the smoak of such a chimney, fall down dead. Cattle, which pasture near to mills, are often killed; and therefore shepherds take great care to keep their sheep at a distance; which, if not by the smoak, must be hurt by the grass, which I often see made blue by the smoak falling on it.'*

Unfortunately, Wilson's recommended treatment, dietary measures and purgation, can only have made matters worse. The unfortunate inhabitants of Leadhills had few other employment opportunities, and it is unlikely that the owner of the mines, the Earl of Hopetoun, would have cared even had he known their plight.

Source: *Occupational Medicine*, Volume 61, Issue 4, June 2011, Page 223, https://doi.org/10.1093/occmed/kqr035. Copyright © The Author 2011.

Reprinted by permission of Oxford University Press on behalf of the Society of Occupational Medicine.

Why I didn't become an occupational physician ...

Alan Bailey

Although I have been a member of the Society of Occupational Medicine (SOM) for at least 30 years, I would never describe myself as an occupational physician. After 5 years of junior jobs in the National Health Service (NHS), I decided I would step off the ladder to consultant physician that my NHS boss was encouraging. I searched the back pages of the *BMJ* and applied for the job of assistant to the Assistant Corporation Medical Advisor (CMA) at the BBC. After 25 min of interrogation from the four doctors, the chairman brought the proceedings to a close with the question 'I see you are a horse person'. This fazed me until I realized he was looking at the interests listed in my CV which included the 'Osler Club'—a London medical history club named after Sir William—nothing to do with ostlers.

I started work in BBC Television Centre in Shepherd's Bush and met real people who were healthy and mostly cleverer and certainly more artistic than me. One of my duties was to examine the sick notes. In the first month, the diagnosis of 'Reiter's disease' appeared three times. When I enquired if the three sufferers knew each other, Personnel had no idea that Reiter's disease was infectious and thought it was related to cramp. It turned out that a woman on the fifth floor was a carrier and two of her consorts had developed arthritis and eye problems as a result of her favours.

I decided to share my excitement by writing it up as a paper about the communication between the medical profession and other disciplines. The CMA turned it down — 'imagine the headlines about venereal disease at the BBC' he said. I then noticed that we had two beds reserved in the local alcoholic unit for our staff but my study on the drinking habits of creative people fared similarly. I next tried stress with the hypothesis that work for cameramen wearing headphones continually receiving instructions from the production gallery was particularly stressful in 'Drama' and 'Outside Broadcast'. I had no control group, but the employment records suggested 'burnout' at an early age. Finally, I measured decibel levels at 'Top of the Pops' and did hearing tests on drummers and Lulu who hit over 100 dBA occasionally. The highest sustained noise levels I measured were in the Television Centre bar between 12.00 and 2.00 p.m. when everyone went for a lunchtime drink!

Needless to say, the CMA was not impressed that I was suggesting that the most respected broadcasting organization in the world was stressing their employees and making them deaf. He showed me an advertisement from the British United Provident Association (BUPA) Medical Centre for a researcher and suggested I apply.

I worked for BUPA for 21 years but it was not real occupational medicine. Nevertheless, in that year at the BBC, I joined the SOM and found that, of all types of physicians, I feel most at home in the company of occupational ones. The SOM allows this mixture and I hope it always will.

Source: *Occupational Medicine*, Volume 58, Issue 5, August 2008, Page 381, https://doi.org/10.1093/occmed/kqm124. Copyright © The Author 2008.

Time to ditch occupational health

Gordon Shepherd

We have all seen the quizzical look on the face of the enquirer at a social event as to what kind of doctor we are when we say *occupational physician*. Neither of these words is well understood and they smack of unnecessary elitism. The first is usually linked with *therapist* and probably, by association, basket weaving and is the second something to do with the science of physics? This is not a good start to a conversation nor is it conducive to a clear understanding in our discourse with the world of business. It is time to ditch *Occupational Health*. Let's call it *Work Medicine* and I would like that we should be called *Work Doctors*. In-house we would be in the *Work Medical Department* and external providers could be *Work Medical Services*. When the Faculty and the Society join up we could look at a dynamic new logo for the *Institute for Work Medicine*. That done, we can now concentrate on attracting new young medical talent to our specialty on the one hand and business users of our services on the other. With regard to the former, we will attract talent if we are glowing from the inside with a new brand and new enthusiasm. But we also need a new direction to capture opportunities lost for both *work medicine* and the businesses we attempt to serve. We must stop telling all and sundry that *work doctors* are expensive. We are not! We add value and a consultation is way cheaper than the 6 weeks' extra sickness absence we have curtailed for the company's employee. Our new branding will hopefully spur us on to communicate better with businesses both collectively and individually. Are we having dialogues with the Confederation of British Industries, the Institute of Directors, the Federation of Small Businesses, the British Chambers of Commerce and the like? (I have been a member of the Policy Council of our local Chamber of Commerce for the last 6 years.) It would be good to reassure these bodies that we can help their corporate members by not being as partisan as our reputation would suggest, by dealing with difficult, occasionally adversarial, situations in an even-handed and balanced manner and generally adding value by, among other things, contributing to the engagement of the employee. We can be more effective if the employers will allow *work medicine* into their systems and a good start would be to send all the incoming Fit Notes directly to *Work Medicine* where a decision can be made about whether and when a return to work consultation takes place. I look forward to there being a better understanding out there as to what we do and I relish my next social event where I will reply, "I am a *work doctor* and I am affiliated to the *Institute for Work Medicine* and you can find us at *inworkmed.com*." Yeah!

Source: *Occupational Medicine*, Volume 63, Issue 7, October 2013, Page 516, https://doi.org/10.1093/occmed/kqt098. Copyright © The Author 2013.

Fifty years ago: 'A new portable hand operated external cardiac compressor'

B.S. Baker

The photographs show details of a portable hand-operated external cardiac compressor which when combined with a simple positive pressure respirator forms a very satisfactory portable heart/lung resuscitator. Previous compressors have required electric power or an oxygen or compressed air supply which makes them less portable, more expensive and more difficult to use correctly. Other hand-operated compressors have been designed for use in hospitals where the patient is static, e.g. in bed. Obviously resuscitation must be continued while the patient is being transported from hazardous conditions as in mines, or fires, or being taken to hospital for defibrillation. This new compressor is cheap, easy to use, cannot over-depress the sternum, and by using a double system of leverage can be used anywhere with the operator in any position relative to the patient. This system of leverage ensures that pressure is transmitted to the patient only. This is an important difference from existing devices where pressure is transmitted to the stretcher thus inflicting up to 10 stones extra pressure on the bearers. This device can be kept wherever respirators such as the 'Ambu' or Porton' are stored, e.g. in mines, ships or ambulances (Figures 105.1 and 105.2).

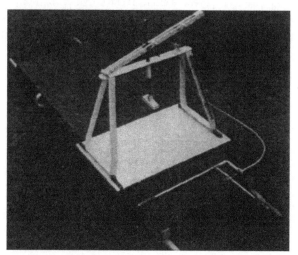

Figure 105.1 Cardiac massage machine.
Reproduced with permission from Baker B. S. (1968). A New Portable Hand Operated External Cardiac Compressor. *Trans Soc Occup Med.* **18**(3):114-5. https://doi.org/10.1093/occmed/18.2.114

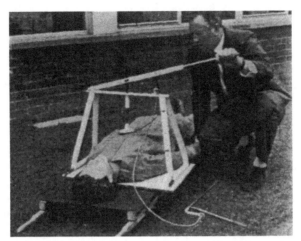

Figure 105.2 Machine in position showing lever extention operation when patient is stationary (i.e. on ambulance).
Reproduced with permission from Baker B. S. (1968). A New Portable Hand Operated External Cardiac Compressor. *Trans Soc Occup Med.* **18**(3):114-5. https://doi.org/10.1093/occmed/18.2.114

Source: *Occupational Medicine*, Volume 68, Issue 7, October 2018, Page 430, https://doi.org/10.1093/occmed/kqx198. © The Author(s) 2018.

Originally from: A new portable hand operated external cardiac compressor. *Trans Soc Occup Med* (1968) 18, 114–115. Available at: *Occup Med (Lond)* 1968; 18:114–115. DOI:10.1093/occmed/18.2.114

Reprinted by permission of Oxford University Press on behalf of the Society of Occupational Medicine.

Tales of Kieran: The occupational physician's odyssey 6—Sniffing about

J.A. Hunter

One of the problems with keeping in touch with Kieran, my occupational physician friend, is that his department is situated in the most inaccessible part of the university. It is hardly a case of just dropping in. You follow a neverending series of fading signs, pointing this way and that to the Occupational Health Department, and eventually arrive at a dilapidated shack that looks as if it should have been condemned some time shortly after the last war. I took this up with Kieran one day over coffee in his department after I had sat outside his office examining the peeling paint and rotting window frames whilst waiting for him to finish an argument with a personnel manager.

'Well, we need to be discreet in our speciality. Our clients don't want everyone seeing them come for appointments. It might be something of a sensitive nature, you know.'

Well, I suppose if you have clients rather than patients then it might be something very sensitive, but I did not voice this to Kieran, who looked as if I had touched on a sore point. I would be surprised if any of his clients ever found the place. But I had also heard recently of some almighty rows in the management committee meetings about the Occupational Health Department, its location and state, particularly since Physics were getting a new building. I had heard there was now a fierce battle going on for the soon-to-be-vacated Physics Department that occupied a prime spot in Chancellor's Court. Furthermore, my spy on the university's management committee had told me that Kieran nearly had an apoplexy when Child Health suggested that Kieran's was one of those Cinderella specialities not deserving of such a prominent location.

A few months later, I realized it had been a few months since I had seen Kieran, so I decided to make the tortuous trip to the boundaries of the campus. He seems to be so involved in so many things that unless I make the effort to keep in contact, I would never see him. Anyway, as I approached, the place looked even more deserted than before, and it was with some surprise that I read a notice on the door which announced that Occupational Health had now relocated to Chancellor's Court. I rushed over and, sure enough, a big sign was being hoisted above the door of the old Physics Department, announcing that it was now Occupational Health. Hardly discreet, I thought, but inside I found Kieran, bent double and wandering around with what looked like a large old radio in his hand, waving it over the bare wooden floorboards.

'What on earth are you doing?', I asked.

'Mercury sniffing', he said without looking up. 'I hit upon the idea when I read about the old Physics Department at Cambridge and how much mercury they discovered under the floorboards when they checked it out. They found kilograms of the stuff. Cost an absolute fortune to remove it all and refurbish the place.'

'And won't they have to do the same here?'

'No. I haven't found any … yet.' Kieran stood up, and I saw the twinkle in his eye. 'Someone sent the Vice Chancellor an account of what happened at Cambridge and she thought it best they didn't move Child Health in here just yet. They said I could have the place whilst we carried out further checks. In the old days, you used to get what you wanted when you had your index finger up the Chief Executive's back passage. These days you have to use your brain.'

He tapped the side of his head knowingly, as the instrument in his hand made a bleeping noise and I saw a needle on a large dial swing frenetically to the right.

'Aaahh, excellent!' Kieran rubbed his hands. 'Found some!'

'But won't you have to move out?'

'Yes, but then we'll get a completely refurbished department', he beamed.

'What about Child Health?'

'Years before the levels settle below safe paediatric levels, absolutely years', and he wandered off happily waving his sniffer. Whilst I am pleased Kieran has got himself a new department, I shall be watching very closely for signs of erythrism in future.

Source: *Occupational Medicine*, Volume 53, Issue 2, March 2003, Page 155, https://doi.org/10.1093/occmed/kqg056. Copyright © Society of Occupational Medicine 2003.

Reprinted by permission of Oxford University Press on behalf of the Society of Occupational Medicine.

One hundred years of the health and safety laboratory 2

Anon

Research into miners' safety lamps was carried out at the Portobello Street Laboratories in Sheffield from the late nineteen twenties (Figure 107.1). At this time, the safety of the lamps was not an issue (as long as they remained undamaged) but the illumination achievable was far from ideal for the workers. The research undertaken looked at design modifications to the lamps and to the mixtures of oils used in them. In addition, the researchers developed a mantle lamp, which was passed to manufacturers to adapt for practical use. Interestingly, the flame safety lamp also helped to detect "firedamp" (the name given to a number of flammable gases, especially methane), and the researchers produced colour photographs to show miners what to look for (a technically complex process at this time).

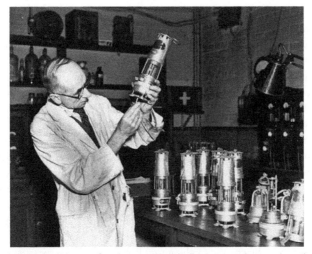

Figure 107.1 Research into miners' safety lamps, Portobello Street Laboratories, Sheffield
© Crown Copyright 2011.

Source: *Occupational Medicine*, Volume 61, Issue 5, August 2011, Page 298, https://doi.org/10.1093/occmed/kqr110. © Crown Copyright 2011.

Reprinted by permission of Oxford University Press on behalf of the Society of Occupational Medicine.

All tied up

John Hobson

It happened a couple of times where I left the house without a tie. Such was my horror at the prospect of seeing patients improperly dressed that I had to buy a tie before the clinic started, once from a supermarket and on the second occasion from a charity shop. The outcome was less than sartorially satisfactory and would not have been good for my colleague or patient feedback. I now keep a selection of suitable neckwear in my car and my record of not having seen a patient, at least outside a surgical environment, without a tie stands. But why wear a tie? Why do male occupational physicians appear so attached to them? Even at meetings and conferences half of us wear one (personal observation). They are, after all, a proven occupational health and safety hazard. They should be removed before entering production environments containing moving machinery. They should not be worn or at least be detachable if there is a risk of assault. They are banned in many clinical environments due to their capacity to act as microbial reservoirs. I remember an office worker colleague getting his tie caught in the shredder and whilst it was eventually hilarious, for a while it wasn't as his head descended towards the revolving metal jaws and his head went puce. He had to be cut free. Even without being garrotted by office equipment, research has shown that wearing a tie raises intraocular pressure, restricts cerebrovascular blood flow and may increase the risk of glaucoma and stroke. Only a fool breaks the two finger rule—can you get two fingers between your collar and your neck? There is some research which shows that how you are dressed has little or no effect on patient satisfaction; in fact other research has shown that patients preferred their general practitioner to be casually dressed. But does this translate to occupational health? There is the expectation and confidence of the employer to be taken into consideration as well as that of the patient (employee) and the employer expects a well-presented service. So this is one of those areas where 'more research is needed', a phrase that *Occupational Medicine* doesn't have the *BMJ*'s luxury of banning. Even without an evidence base, this is yet another disease for which being male and getting older are the main and perhaps only risk factors. At the Bear Inn in Oxford, the walls are famously adorned by the amputated ends of more than 4500 ties. The former landlord, Alan Course, began the tradition in 1952 in between working as a cartoonist at the Oxford Mail. He used scissors to collect ties he didn't have in his collection. In exchange the donor received half a pint of bitter although it isn't stated whether the donor was always willing or compliant. Maybe the forthcoming Royal College of Occupational Health should initiate a similar scheme and the occupational physician's personal occupational health and safety hazard can finally be eradicated?

Source: *Occupational Medicine*, Volume 64, Issue 5, July 2014, Page 316, https://doi.org/10.1093/occmed/kqu012. © The Author 2014.

Reprinted by permission of Oxford University Press on behalf of the Society of Occupational Medicine.

Why I became an occupational physician …

Simon E. Asogwa

I lost 3 years of my training because of the Nigerian Civil War (1967–70) being on the Biafran side. Consequently, when the war ended, I was keen on pursuing a course that would enable me to 'catch up' with my colleagues on the Nigerian side. My initial choice was medical jurisprudence. I had read Keith Simpson's book on the subject as an undergraduate and a combination of medical and legal knowledge excited me. With the DMJ, I believed, I would have rapid professional and academic growth. I wrote to Simpson who invited me to his department for training. With this offer, I obtained a federal government scholarship. On arrival at Guy's Hospital in the severe winter of October 1971, I met Simpson who explained to me that I would first have to obtain the MRCP in pathology before proceeding to the DMJ. I had not bargained for that and that was the last I saw of him.

I got a job as a casualty officer at St Stephen's Hospital, Chelsea. While there I read an advertisement in the *British Medical Journal* on the occupational medicine course at the London School of Hygiene and Tropical Medicine. I applied and was offered a place and on one of my free days I visited the school. On arrival, I met the director of the Institute of Occupational Health, R. S. F. Schilling. During what turned out to be an interview, he inquired about my background and especially my industrial medical experience. Of course I had none, having just come out of a civil war. Two days later, to my utter dismay, I received a letter withdrawing the offer! However, I would still be accepted on condition that I first obtained an admission for the diploma in Tropical Public Health (DTPH) at the Ross Institute. I blamed myself for that visit to the Institute of Occupational Health.

It was only later that I realized that the visit was a blessing in disguise. I passed the DTPH, reapplied and was offered a place for the MSc in 1973. My lecturers included Malcolm Harrington and Suzette Gauvain. To enable me to have some industrial medical exposure, the institute arranged attachments with the National Coal Board with F. Halliwell and with British Airways at Heathrow Airport.

On returning to Nigeria in December 1974, I was employed as a lecturer and consultant occupational and community physician at the University of Nigeria Teaching Hospital. I also had a part-time appointment at the Nigersteel Company. With my training in tropical public health and occupational medicine and having the experience of practising both simultaneously, I felt there was a need for a book on the practice of occupational medicine in a developing country like Nigeria. Consequently, I wrote *A Guide to Occupational Health Practice in Developing Countries* principally for my medical students and residents. The book was prefaced by Mustafa Khogali, then of the Institute of Occupational Health and the third edition has recently been published in 2007.

Source: *Occupational Medicine*, Volume 58, Issue 6, September 2008, Page 450, https://doi.org/10.1093/occmed/kqn036. Copyright © The Author 2008.

Reprinted by permission of Oxford University Press on behalf of the Society of Occupational Medicine.

Fashion victims

Paul Grime

As occupational health professionals, we may be fashion leaders or followers, or just people who buy and wear clothes, but we probably do not give much thought to where and how our clothes are made. And, are we aware of the hidden price for garment workers in developing countries such as Bangladesh?

In April 2013, 1129 people were killed and 2500 injured when a garment factory collapsed at the Rana Plaza complex in Dhaka, Bangladesh. More than half the victims were women and some were children. This was the deadliest garment factory accident in history. A government inquiry found that the reasons for the collapse included poor construction materials, corrupt building practices, vibrating industrial equipment at the top of a commercial building and people being forced into an unsafe structure. A recent editorial in this journal highlighted the costs of cheap fashion for workers in the garment manufacturing industry [1].

On 5 September 2013, the Church of Bangladesh Group (including Anglican Alliance, Church Mission Society, Church of Scotland, Council for World Mission, Diocese of Llandaff, Methodist Church in Britain, Oxford Mission and United Society) launched a campaign calling for global justice, wage justice and living justice for Bangladeshi garment workers [2]. Consumers are urged to consider what conditions are like for people who make their clothes, and to write to retailers and suppliers to ask:

1. Does your company import clothing made in Bangladesh or other developing countries?
2. Do you set minimum workplace standards for your suppliers?
3. Do you ensure they pay their workers a fair wage?
4. Does your company support the international Accord on Fire and Building Safety?
5. What assessments have you made recently of your supply chain to ensure significant and sustained improvements in the working conditions of garment workers?

Other suggestions include:

- Writing to members of the UK and European parliaments to ask for representations to be made to the retailers selling garments made in Bangladesh, and also to the Bangladeshi Government to improve conditions for workers in the industry.
- Talking to trade bodies to put pressure on the Bangladesh Garment Manufacturers and Exporters Association and the Bangladesh Knitting Manufacturers and Exports Association.
- Meeting the owners or managers of shops that sell clothes imported from Bangladesh.

The key points in the campaign include:

- Security for workers, protection from fire and unhygienic conditions in the factories, keeping factory gates open with guards during working hours.
- Facilities on-site for infants and babies of women garment workers and health facilities for pregnant garment workers.

- Canteen facilities for lunch and breaks, holidays, sick leave.
- An industry-wide forum to work with government to improve industry standards.

This is an international occupational health and safety issue of monumental proportions. It is also a matter of social justice. In response to acknowledging the nature and the scale of the problem, and our collective responsibility to prevent occupational morbidity and mortality in the garment manufacturing industry, here is a campaign that occupational health and safety professionals should consider supporting.

References

1. **Hobson J.** To die for? The health and safety of fast fashion. *Occup Med (Lond)* 2013;**63**:317–319.
2. http://www.methodist.org.uk/mission/world-church/asia-pacific/bangladesh/new-justice-for-bangladesh (6 October 2013, date last accessed).

Source: *Occupational Medicine*, Volume 64, Issue 1, January 2014, Page 66, https://doi.org/10.1093/occmed/kqt133. Copyright © The Author 2013.

One hundred years of the health and safety laboratory 3

Anon

This picture (Figure 111.1) shows staff heaving the cannon into the coal dust explosion test area on the Buxton site in the 1920s. These explosions took place in a number of galleries, but this picture shows the cannon used in the largest gallery. Coal dust was ignited by firing the cannon charged with 790g of gunpowder stemmed with 20cm of fine dry coal dust. The cannon was placed 12m from the closed end of the gallery, and pointed into a tube some 1m in diameter and 3.1m long, along which 9.1kg of coal dust was scattered. The coal used was crushed so that 85% passed through a sieve with 200meshes to every 2.54cm. This experiment was demonstrated at the opening of the Buxton site on 14 June 1927 to visitors including the Viscount Chelmsford, who was Chairman of the miners welfare committee, and Colonel the Rt Hon G R Lane Fox, Secretary for Mines.

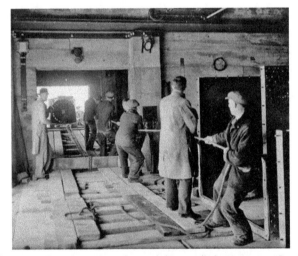

Figure 111.1 Staff heaving the cannon into the coal dust explosion test area, Buxton 1920s
© Crown Copyright 2011.

Source: *Occupational Medicine*, Volume 61, Issue 5, August 2011, Page 334, https://doi.org/10.1093/occmed/kqr109. © Crown copyright 2011.

Fifty years ago: 'Malaises and Discontents'

Anon

Fourteen working days were lost in 1962 for every insured person, a total of nearly 300 million working days. Sickness benefit payments cost the State £160 million, about one-sixth of the total expenditure on the National Health Service. 9 ¼ million new claims were made for sickness benefit in 1963, an increase of over 2 million over the 1950 figure. These are some of the many facts given in a recent publication by the Office of Health Economics. The increase both in days lost and in spells commencing is partly accounted for by an increase in the total number of insured persons. The male working population increased by 0.8 per cent per year from 1953-4; the female decreased by 1.2 per cent per year, but the preponderance of men in the insured population meant a slight increase in the total each year. Even when allowance is made for this, and for the effect of ageing, however, the number both of working days lost and of spells commencing was substantially higher than in 1953, for both sexes. There has been a change in the pattern of causes of incapacity: absences from respiratory tuberculosis, skin diseases, rheumatism and peptic ulcer have shown a striking decline, and those due to injuries and accidents, 'debility', vascular lesions, psychoneurosis, psychosis and bronchitis an increase. Bronchitis remains the principal cause of lost time in men.

Some of the facts set out, and trends shown, may not be particularly significant, but others at least suggest the kind of questions we should be asking about our society. For instance, we know the cost of ill health to the Exchequer, but what does it cost industry in addition—not only in payments under sick pay schemes, when these exist, but in idle machinery and lost orders, or alternatively in bigger labour forces than should be required to maintain production? The plain fact is that most industrial managements do not know, and those who are least informed tend also to regard expenditure on occupational health services as a luxury they cannot afford. Measures of compulsion are not incompatible with a 'free society', as the whole history of our factory legislation shows, in spite of the screams of the die-hards who swear each social advance will mean their ruin. The issue is basically an economic one, and will ultimately have to be faced without sentimentality or deference to sectional interests. Why do people go sick? The answer 'because they are ill' is tautological unless 'illness' is given a much wider connotation than it has in everyday speech. It is common knowledge that a host of extraneous factors determine whether a person who does not feel very well takes the day off work. A correspondent recently sent us a note on a small personal study suggesting that the state of the weather and the incidence of pay-day were among these. Undoubtedly feelings of worth, responsibility and job satisfaction are others, and when these are lacking, absence attributed to frankly psychological causes, and to 'debility' as well as to some somatic causes will tend to rise.

Source: *Occupational Medicine*, Volume 65, Issue 5, July 2015, Page 401, https://doi.org/10.1093/occmed/kqv033. Copyright © The Author 2015.

Originally from: Malaises and Discontents. Available at: *Occup Med (Lond)* 1965;15:81–82.

Reprinted by permission of Oxford University Press on behalf of the Society of Occupational Medicine.

Why I became an occupational physician …

Clodagh Cashman

'The farther backward you can look, the farther forward you are likely to see' (Winston Churchill).

When I was younger, I travelled the countryside with my father, a veterinary surgeon somewhat in the manner of 'All Creatures Great and Small'. It was essential to explore the nature of the question of illness in its context and to listen to the people involved. Perhaps this served to focus my interests and fit with a career in medicine? Rather than veterinary medicine, it seemed to provide a sensible opportunity to avoid the harsher physical environment, e.g. cold outdoor duties, at 3.00 a.m., without light. This flawed logic was quickly revealed during internship and underpinned by the lure of patients towards George Clooney's caring doctor on 'ER' and away from my medical ministrations. Had I read Shem's 'House of God' circulating in early training who knows what career would have resulted …?

Medical residency in the USA provided an opportunity to train in the multicultural learning organization in the Midwest and felt more like working in the United Nations. Questions constantly came to mind while taking care of patients about preventing illness. Broadening options with a master's degree in public health medicine made sense. After all, Snow's 19th century intervention on the Broad Street pump handle prevented cholera and helped numbers of people without a hospital. And the context-specific opportunity in the work setting came to me on a community immunization programme. Illness interventions could occur outside the hospital setting not only in a primary care clinic but also … in the workplace.

'It's the economy stupid …' Political phrase

Training in occupational medicine followed and you may ask why, given broader economic uncertainties. Encounters with colleagues with great compassion, skill and common sense and even better a great sense of humour reveal that 'it's the people stupid …' when it comes to enjoying work. The training programme (in Ireland) supported adjunctive opportunities as a trainee representative to UEMS Occupational Medicine Section, an elective with the US Preventive Service Task Force and with the Cochrane Injuries Group. Skills and expertise were gathered that facilitate my work today.

Career guidance was limited in the carbolic corridors of hospital as an intern. When you think about it though, what specialist is best placed to work on questions as diverse as health effects and nanotechnology or deep-sea exploration or high-altitude engineering? Or hearing protection programmes from brass bands to U2? Or devise global health strategy and malaria protection for international workers? Or evaluating the nature of a pilot's experience in relation to a doctor's?

There are as many health questions to be considered in the workplace, as there are workers; to the expert level of not attributing an individual's circumstance to a medical cause when other factors are at play. In relation to choosing an interesting career with excellent mentors outside the hospital setting, if I was asked about doing it again—to quote from the final sentence in James Joyce's 'Ulysses'— 'I said yes I will Yes'.

Source: *Occupational Medicine*, Volume 58, Issue 8, December 2008, Page 533, https://doi.org/10.1093/occmed/kqn114. Copyright © The Author 2008.

Reprinted by permission of Oxford University Press on behalf of the Society of Occupational Medicine.

The Ontario Workplace Health Champions programme

D. Linn Holness and Gary Liss

Incorporating occupational health content into the medical school curriculum is an ongoing challenge. In 1994, the Ontario Medical Association Section of Occupational and Environmental Medicine gathered together groups with an interest in clinical workplace health including government, universities, hospitals, research organizations and organized labour. A needs assessment was conducted and documented gaps in knowledge, skills and training related to workplace health. An occupational medicine physician (G.L.) was appointed and funded through a provincial educational project, the Physician Education Project in Workplace Health. The Workplace Safety and Insurance Board (WSIB) undertook a survey that documented the lack of educational activities in several of the five medical schools in Ontario. As a result of the needs assessment and survey of medical schools, the WSIB developed the Workplace Health Champions Program (WHCP).

The WHCP supports Ontario medical schools to enhance and expand their curricula in occupational health. Starting in 1999 the five (and then six) medical faculties in Ontario signed agreements with the WSIB agreeing to: (i) develop and implement a workplace health curriculum to support medical training in workplace health issues primarily at the undergraduate education level, (ii) select a physician as Workplace Health Champion (WHC) to assist in the development and implementation of a workplace curriculum, (iii) keep the WSIB informed of the progress and impacts of the curriculum in the training programme and (iv) participate with the WSIB in an evaluation of the curriculum and its impact on the training of new physicians.

The medical school selects the WHC in collaboration with the WSIB. The champions are usually occupational medicine specialists or family physicians with a practice in occupational medicine. The WSIB provides financial support to the school to help support the champion and their work.

The champions work with the medical education and curriculum committees in their schools to identify places for occupational health content, either as sessions specifically devoted to occupational health or in other sessions such as case studies. They also offer opportunities for electives and research projects. One school is in the process of developing a video to demonstrate occupational history taking.

The six champions, an external academic advisor (D.L.H.) and the WSIB occupational disease medical director and vice president health services meet twice a year. These meetings provide an opportunity for the champions to support each other and share their experiences and resources. The WHCs recognize the challenges inherent in integrating workplace health into medical curricula. The champions worked to develop a core set of curriculum content and identify key resources.

Evaluation is an important component of the programme. Evaluation has focussed on process measures such as the activities and number of hours of workplace health training. The group has developed a core set of examination questions that can be used by the champions. One school has included specific questions on the student examination and can report student performance on workplace health content. The group is developing several objective structured clinical exam stations which can be used for evaluation.

Source: *Occupational Medicine*, Volume 64, Issue 6, September 2014, Page 447, https://doi.org/10.1093/occmed/kqu090. Copyright © The Author 2014.

Going through the motions

Mike Gibson

The measurement of deep body temperature in pilots is necessary to determine the thermal load arising from a combination of environmental factors, workload and clothing insulation, mitigated by cabin and personal conditioning systems. In the USA, this was usually achieved by measuring rectal temperatures. Royal Air Force (RAF) pilots are generally less amenable. At the RAF Institute of Aviation Medicine, we had been using ear canal temperatures (T_{ac}) but the risk of mishap caused by dislodging the probe whilst flying at high speed and low level was significant.

One of our technicians therefore developed a radio-pill, based on the one invented by Prof. Heinz Wolff to measure intestinal pressures. To investigate how the measurements from this pill compared with those from the ear canal, oesophagus and rectum, I devised an experiment to drive deep body temperatures up and down as fast as possible. After being suitably instrumented, the subject entered a bath at 42°C until T_{ac} reached 38.5°C. He then leapt into a bath filled with water at 10°C and remained there until T_{ac} reached 35°C before returning to the hot bath.

These were the days before ethics committees and we relied on a process of reciprocal consent: 'I'll be a subject in your unpleasant experiment if you'll be a subject in mine.' Common practice was for the experimental leader to carry out the pilot study. The first question that crossed our minds was the impact on blood pressure. In my pilot run, my systolic and diastolic pressures peaked transiently at >300/200 mmHg just after entering the cold bath. We were all young, fit and healthy so, as there were other things to concentrate on, we did not measure blood pressure in the actual experiment.

The experience was as unpleasant as expected. What we did not expect, however, was that four of the six experimental subjects described a feeling of intense disorientation, of tumbling forwards, just after entering the cold bath. One brave soul repeated the experience in the dark and we obtained an infrared film of his vertical nystagmus. He was the only subject not to swear on entering the cold water but he did shout 'Ow' repeatedly. We later explained the phenomenon as a result of reinforcing convection currents being generated in the vertical semicircular canals, the currents in the horizontal canals cancelling each other out.

In terms of the primary purpose of the experiment, the temperature and the rate of change of temperature measured in the gastrointestinal tract was about halfway between the measurements in the oesophagus and rectum. The really unpleasant bit was retrieving the pills afterwards for recalibration.

Source: *Occupational Medicine*, Volume 65, Issue 4, June 2015, Page 295, https://doi.org/10.1093/occmed/kqu104. Copyright © The Author 2015.

How to learn science

Anthony Seaton

What first fired your enthusiasm for medicine? I suspect it was not school teaching of science; more likely, I think in most cases it was a vague feeling of altruism. I confess that the basic sciences of medicine were something of a chore for me, and only when I started to study pathology and see patients did I find learning medicine really exciting. So when the new curriculum came along in the 1990s, I welcomed the opportunity to help introduce it in my Medical School. By the time I retired, eight generations of students had graduated without the intensive learning of the basic sciences that I had been subjected to but, we hoped, with a better integrated understanding of health and illness. Are they better or worse than we were? We shall never know, as the chance for comparison has been missed. All we can do is compare us with them, and there is a certain bias in this! How can we compare ourselves, with that accumulation of guile, confidence, experience, selective memory and self-delusion that we might characterize as wisdom, with young graduates coming through the system now? They seem raw, but in a moment of realism most will remember with embarrassment how raw we were at that stage.

I was reminded of this when the English Secretary of State for Education proposed a 'back to basics' move in the school science curriculum, including such fundamental matters as Newton's laws of thermodynamics. Yes! It was quickly pointed out that he was confusing motion with hot air and so many centuries out that he might benefit from a bit of scientific understanding himself. Behind his suggestion seemed to lie a belief that teaching science based on climate change is getting it the wrong way round, the implication being that if children understood scientific principles they would realize that the story of climate change is probably eyewash. Which way round is better?

An historical look at climate change shows how easily it may be used to introduce children (and indeed adults including the administrative stream of the civil service and politicians) to basic science in a way that attracts and holds interest. Why is the earth warming? Greenhouse gases. What are they and how are they made? Chemistry. Why do they make the earth warmer? Physics. How may we control their rise? The carbon and nitrogen cycles—biology. How do we understand the effects? Mathematical statistics. How do we try to understand causation? Philosophy of science. And it doesn't stop there: how did these ideas develop? History. What are the possible consequences? Economics and human geography. How should we deal with the issues? Politics. Science is about asking questions and trying to find answers.

I could go on but, in short, it is difficult to think of a more interesting way to introduce anyone, of any age or level of sophistication, to the fundamental concepts of science and to their implications for all of us.

Source: *Occupational Medicine*, Volume 61, Issue 8, December 2011, Page 582, https://doi.org/10.1093/occmed/kqr123. Copyright © The Author 2011.

Reprinted by permission of Oxford University Press on behalf of the Society of Occupational Medicine.

Why I became an occupational physician …

Timothy P. Finnegan

Of the hundreds of ward rounds, clinics, lectures, tutorials and operations that you attended at medical school, which do you remember? One that strongly influenced me was a ward round by Prof. Pat Lawther of the Barts Air Pollution Unit. He cultivated the image of the archetypal 'mad professor' and spoke passionately about the importance and relevance of the jobs done by the in-patients being cared for.

By the time I qualified in 1975, I had developed a strong inclination towards prevention. Thus, instead of becoming a third-generation general practitioner or going into one of the hospital spe-cialities I enjoyed, I stuck to my beliefs and looked at openings in preventive medicine. Then, the National Health Service was not much involved with prevention but I knew the army was. I enquired during my final year and the army was very welcoming and looked like fun as well. One result was that I did my house physician's job at the Queen Alexandra's Military Hospital, Millbank. The inpatient soldiers who were being discharged into civilian life from there reinforced my interest in the links between ill-health and work.

At that time, the army had a speciality called 'Army Health'. This required Diplomas in Tropical Medicine and Hygiene, Industrial Health and Public Health. I started this training in 1979 but very soon Army Health was reorganized because of the development of the Faculties of Public Health Medicine and Occupational Medicine. I chose the latter and consequently in 1983, I had the priv-ilege of being the first person in the army to take the Associate of the Faculty of Occupational Medicine examination.

The strong links between the army's health care organization and its overall management (chain of command) clearly showed me that it was essential to do some leadership and manage-ment training. I was fortunately successful in the necessary examinations and attended The Staff College, Camberley in 1985.

The Armed Forces view work as one of the desirable outcomes of health care, as Dame Carol Black has recently noted in Working for a Healthier Tomorrow. This strong connection between health and health care gives the army some unusual characteristics. First, there are very strong ties between general practitioners and occupational physicians. Second, all health care personnel are very aware of the importance of returning people to work. As an occupational physician, all this is very attractive. I decided that the army was an excellent place to work and so it has proved. The added opportunities to become a major line manager of medical assets have been a bonus.

Returning to my beginning, the lesson I draw from all this is that we must continue to press the importance of occupational health in the undergraduate curriculum. The benefits to the UK from linking health care, work and their importance to society are becoming increasingly clear. It is an important task for us.

Source: *Occupational Medicine*, Volume 59, Issue 3, May 2009, Page 207, https://doi.org/10.1093/occmed/kqp008. Copyright © The Author 2009.

Reprinted by permission of Oxford University Press on behalf of the Society of Occupational Medicine.

Hammerfest: Occupational medicine at 70° north

Emma Hirons

At 70° north and 600 miles above the Arctic Circle, the tiny Norwegian port of Hammerfest is the world's northernmost town. Funding from the Faculty of Occupational Medicine (Mobbs Student Elective Fellowship) and the Nuffield Department of Population Health (Eoin Hodgson Memorial Bursary) gave me the opportunity to learn about occupational medicine in the Arctic. I was able to see and compare a very modern industry with the centuries old traditional occupation of reindeer husbandry which exist side by side.

In 2007, Norwegian company Statoil began processing liquid natural gas (LNG) from the Snøhvit gas field at the Melkøye plant in Hammerfest. Natural gas extracted from the seabed is piped to Melkøye for processing. With no surface installations, Snøhvit is a completely unmanned offshore installation, monitored and controlled from Melkøye. Since workers occasionally visit Snøhvit, Melkøye is classed as both an onshore and offshore development and must satisfy the different health and safety requirements of each location. Natural gas is processed at −162°C, so employees must wear gloves and hard hats to avoid cold injuries and head injuries from falling icicles from overhead apparatus. Strict rules govern how long offshore employees can work outside depending on temperature and wind chill factor. Activities in uncomfortable positions or with raised arms to reach overhead controls predispose to musculoskeletal pain affecting the shoulders, neck and back so occupational health physicians are included in design teams to improve ergonomics. Gas leaks are a potentially catastrophic hazard. Employees carry gas masks and Melkøye is trialling a new system for more accurate detection of poisonous by-products. Melkøye, Hammerfest hospital and the emergency services run catastrophe training to ensure that protocols are in place in the event of a disaster.

The Sami are an indigenous northern Scandinavian population, traditionally reindeer herders, with their own culture and language. Reindeer husbandry follows a strict calendar. During winter reindeer graze inland. In April, the Sami round up the herd into a fence (pen) using snowmobiles. Each family collects their reindeer from the main herd by dragging the animal by the antlers into the family fence. The herds travel to coastal grazing areas over summer. Reindeer herders are twice as likely to die from work-related accidents than other occupations in the region [1]. All herders fear penetrating eye injury from an antler, but eye protection is not used. Fixing the fence requires bare fingers, so the Sami put their hands inside their jackets every 5min to avoid frostbite. Although an integral part of their work, snowmobiles can cause significant trauma due to powerful, heavy modern vehicles and avalanches.

Whereas Statoil is committed to continually assessing and improving working conditions, the Sami do not have occupational health and continue to work as they have for centuries. There is a campaign to recognize traditional Sami occupations as a degree subject. This would be a good platform from which to educate them about occupational health and to work alongside the Sami to ensure that health and safety alterations in traditional trades are acceptable.

Reference

1. **Daerga L, Edin-Liljegren A, Sjölander P.** Work-related musculoskeletal pain among reindeer herding Sami in Sweden—a pilot study on causes and prevention. *Int J Circumpolar Health* 2004;**63**(Suppl. 2):343–348.

Source: *Occupational Medicine*, Volume 64, Issue 8, December 2014, Page 628, https://doi.org/10.1093/occmed/kqu132. Copyright © The Author 2014.

Fifty years ago: 'Height, Weight and Obesity in an Industrial Population'

R.W. Howell

In introducing their paper, 'Heights and Weights of Business Men', May and Wright (1961) pointed out that the height and weight tables commonly used in this country are based on American 1912 Life Insurance tables. More use is currently made of tables based on data from the nineteen-twenties, but with the vast social and dietary changes which have occurred in the past three decades, these, too, may well be in need of reappraisal.

The present sample consisted of over 2000 males employed at the UK Atomic Energy Authority's establishment at Windscale and Calder, in Cumberland. This site not only houses the four Magnox reactors at Calder Hall, and the Advanced Gas Reactor (A.G.R.), but has also a large chemical processing plant; in addition, research in several fields is undertaken there. Most of the manual workers are natives of the area, whereas the non-manual staff tend to be from widely scattered parts of the country. Of the males employed, some two-thirds are manual workers. A large proportion of the manual staff consists of general and process workers, but there are large numbers of craftsmen and their mates, plus over 200 craft apprentices. Among the non-manual staff, there are scientists, engineers, technical officers, administrative and clerical officers, together with a wide range of other supporting staff.

Although the relationship between obesity and high mortality has been well documented, largely because of the initial interest and available material of the American insurance companies (Medical Impairment Study, 1931) (Dublin, 1953: Dublin and Marks, 1951), not a great deal has been written of the effect of obesity on sickness absence rates.

A review of 1963 sickness absence for this Windscale sample showed that there was no significant difference in the rates for the normal, the underweight and the grossly overweight groups. This would appear to be because happily serious illness constitutes such a small proportion of total sickness absence in industry. Certainly the overweight group had an excess of episodes for heart diseases, gastroenteritis, dyspepsia (but not gastritis), genitourinary illness, bone and joint disease, influenza and bronchitis. But the numbers were too small, in a single year, for this to be regarded as significant. The normal weight group, not unexpectedly perhaps, had a higher ratio of peptic ulcer cases. Those 10% or more underweight had a high incidence of gastroenteritis and peptic ulcer, but slightly fewer accidents than were expected.

Heights, weights, ages and degree of obesity for a sample of just over 2000 males in an industrial population have been recorded and analyzed. Comparisons have been made with some aspects of previous surveys by Kemsley, and by May and Wright. There is some confirmation that average heights and weights have increased since the commencement of Kemsley's survey in 1943. Comparisons have been made of certified sickness absence in the sample when these men have been classified by degree of obesity. Probably the high proportion found to be 20 per cent or more overweight poses an eventual health problem, the extent of which is not perhaps generally recognized, in view of the increased mortality to which these subjects are liable. Two per cent of the sample had glycosuria of unknown aetiology.

Source: *Occupational Medicine*, Volume 65, Issue 6, August 2015, Page 458, https://doi.org/10.1093/occmed/kqv034. Copyright © The Author 2015.

Originally from: Height, Weight and Obesity in an Industrial Population. *Trans Ass Industr Med Offrs* (1965) 15, 25. Available at: *Occup Med (Lond)* 1965;**15**:25–28. DOI:10.1093/occmed/15.1.25.

The raincoat sign

John Hobson

She was wearing the most fluorescent raincoat I think I have ever seen but I already knew from our previous meeting that the consultation was likely to be interesting. She had initially been referred by her manager, who was concerned by her behaviour, and at that first appointment she had announced her presence to all and sundry by demanding to know very loudly who I was when I invited her to come through from the waiting room. At the end of that consultation we had fortunately agreed that she was unfit to work and I had written to the general practitioner expressing my concerns about her mental state. Those prior concerns were confirmed at the second consultation where, despite informing me after 5min that she didn't wish to proceed, I was still trying to terminate the consultation an hour later. She grabbed the copy of my letter to the GP, annotated it with what can only be described as violent flourishes of a pencil and then refused to let me have it back before ripping it up in my face. She spontaneously reassured me that she was unlikely to become physically aggressive; I wasn't convinced. How could I accuse her of delusional infestational paranoia she demanded? I couldn't because it wasn't a term I had used or even heard of. When she finally stormed out of the consultation room it was only to continue shouting and gesticulating in the waiting area. She finally announced she was going for a walk despite an on-going downpour of monsoon proportions and the lack of any convincing waterproofing protection apart from her very short but bright raincoat. There was relief mixed with apprehension for the whole department when she returned half an hour later and finally drove away. I rang the GP to further express my concerns and then her manager to suggest her professional body was contacted. Some patients announce themselves by their accessories: the tinted glasses, the cervical collar, the crutches, the walking stick. Some, like the collar, seem to have gone out of fashion, discredited by lack of evidence. Others are acceptable; a randomized control trial of walking sticks in osteoarthritis of the knee has shown them to be of significant benefit in pain reduction and improved mobility. But what about the delusional woman and her fluorescent raincoat? Would she normally wear something like that? She wouldn't normally behave like that so perhaps it is a clinical sign? The detection of delusion in the occupational health clinic is rarely straightforward; some patients present on-going and long-term conundrums, tolerated by their communities, workplaces and general practitioners, often for decades as it is easier to accept them as just strange rather than upsetting the apple cart. They resist medication unless there is a true crisis and then stop taking it once better so the cycle repeats. The last I heard my delusional lady had returned to normal but not to work as she refused to see occupational health.

Source: *Occupational Medicine*, Volume 64, Issue 6, September 2014, Page 453, https://doi.org/10.1093/occmed/kqu015. Copyright © The Author 2014.

Why I became an occupational physician …

W. Glass

In January 1958, my wife and I embarked on the Port Hobart in Wellington, New Zealand, bound for London, she a fare paying passenger, and I the ship's doctor in this 12-passenger cargo vessel. I was young, impetuous and impatient.

Looking back now it was my first occupational medicine job—noise and asbestos in the engine room, sunstroke for the ship's captain and gonorrhoea for the crew. We arrived at the London dockside with our bags, looked at each other and laughed. No job, nowhere to live, and not a lot of money, but one contact—Dr Chris Wood, Senior Lecturer in Occupational Health at the London School of Hygiene and Tropical Medicine.

A phone call to Chris led to a visit, an offer of board at their home in Swiss Cottage and in a few weeks after watching my unsuccessful attempts to get a hospital job, a suggestion that 'occupational medicine is the coming speciality, Bill'. Chris arranged for me to meet Professor Walton, Public Health, who after some surprise at my brief (1 year) medical experience said, 'oh well, young fellow, you are here now so we had better enrol you in the DPH course'. As the course was not starting till later in the year, he kindly found a job for me at the Southend-on-Sea Local Health Authority.

The London School was exciting, with such teachers as Richard Schilling, Tom Garland (who had been Director of Industrial Hygiene in New Zealand for 10 years), Donald Hunter, Bradford Hill, Richard Doll, Professors Walton, Crowder, Spooner and McDonald in Public Health and always Chris as guide and mentor. Then, there were the weekly evening lectures—Jonas Salk and Karl Evang were two I remember—and of course politics, tennis, music and the theatre.

Cheddi Jagan had been deposed as elected Prime Minister of British Guiana and come to London to plead his case. Maria Callas and Joan Sutherland were singing at Covent Garden—we queued for two days and two nights for tickets! Oistrakh and Glen Gould at the Festival Hall and Menuhin at the Albert Hall. Brendon Behan's Borstal Boy playing at the theatre and Rod Laver lost his first Wimbledon final—these memories are still so clear.

The last 51 years in occupational medicine have gone too quickly, have been fun and an adventure. Unexpected highlights have included 6 years on the International Commission on Occupational Health Board, an invitation to give the James Smiley Lecture in Dublin at the Irish Faculty, and being linked with David Ferguson in Australia in the Annual Ferguson-Glass Oration at the Australasian Faculty Annual Meetings.

Occupational medicine continues to excite and remains a passion as I still spend 40 plus hours a week in the specialty—still listening to the workers' experience and still trying to put into practice the principles taught by such great teachers at the London School of Hygiene and Tropical Medicine over 50 years ago.

Source: *Occupational Medicine*, Volume 59, Issue 7, October 2009, Page 446, https://doi.org/10.1093/occmed/kqp105. Copyright © The Author 2009.

The art of observation

Karen Coomer

For it may safely be said, not that the habit of ready and correct observation will by itself make us useful nurses, but that without it we shall be useless with all our devotion.

Florence Nightingale
Notes on Nursing: What it is and what it is not
(1860), 160

It's almost the end of a typical case management day, one more referral to see. The room is hot and stuffy and my mind wanders to the challenges of the motorway traffic ahead. My last referral arrives—a gentleman in his early 30s originally from sub-Saharan Africa, one of many migrant workers in this work environment. He works on the production line in the factory; it's a mix of physical and repetitive work requiring the ability to be able to pack boxes and then hand-ball them onto pallets at the end of the line. He works a three shift pattern and I see from the referral form that he favours working nights and regularly volunteers to work overtime. I launch into the usual occupational health introductory speech but he looks down at the table in front of us and declines to take off his woolly hat and coat. He has recently been in hospital for 5 days and has had sporadic absence for infections, a fit note states he has had a viral infection. He reports he does not know what is wrong with him but tells me he feels very well now; it sounds a well-rehearsed impassive speech from a gaunt looking face. He looks up and I see fear in his eyes, he looks away and I put the referral form to one side. We chat about his time in the UK and slowly he uncrosses his arms, he tells me he supports family in the UK and an extended family back in Africa. I get the picture—he needs his job and ill health is not on his personal agenda. There is an elephant in the room; we both know it needs to be discussed. When I mention the virus he lowers his eyes, then looks out the window and stays silent for a long few moments. I share the silence with him. He then makes eye contact and I sense he is not ready to discuss it. I ask if I can contact his specialist for further information, he looks relieved and we discuss the next steps. He takes off his hat and I slowly feel the rapport building between us, we finish the consultation and he offers to shake my hand. I will be seeing him again. I drive home and reflect on my day, thankful that my last referral wasn't a telephone assessment.

Source: *Occupational Medicine*, Volume 65, Issue 1, January 2015, Page 71, https://doi.org/10.1093/occmed/kqu148. Copyright © The Author 2015.
Reprinted by permission of Oxford University Press on behalf of the Society of Occupational Medicine.

Worst job ads from history—situation vacant plague doctor

Kirstie Gibson

An exciting public health opportunity has arisen in the City of London. Due to a recent vacancy, the infectious diseases team are looking for a full- or part-time plague doctor [1]. Applicants must be qualified physicians and preferably members of the College of Physicians. Apothecaries need not apply.

Working with a team of seekers and watchers, the jobholder will admit patients to pest houses and attend patients in their own homes. They will be expected to record disease statistics for the Bills of Mortality [2], examine patients safely at a distance, perform post mortems on an occasional basis, follow infection control plague orders, take details of wills and testaments, and give lifestyle advice for the afterlife.

The role includes the requirement to maintain strict quarantine regulations and not to attend public gatherings. Physicians must carry a white stick to indicate their professional status to the public [3].

The Corporation may pay some expenses including disinfectant fumigants, lozenges and a small allowance for a supply of 'sack' (fortified sweet wine [4]) for medicinal and preventive purposes only. Applicants must be fully fit and possess a valid certificate of health. Witnessed and vouchsafed evidence of survival of a previous attack of the deadly pestilence is a distinct advantage and will be looked upon very favourably [5].

Applicants must understand that the role involves long periods of social exclusion and solitude. The City cannot accept responsibility for the illness or death of the successful applicant, as it is generally public knowledge that death rates are currently running at between 15 and 60% in some areas [6] and treatment and prevention have not yet been discovered.

For further information and advice on this challenging but well-recompensed career opportunity please contact experienced and well-respected senior plague physicians Dr Nathaniel Hodges [7] or Dr Thomas Witherly [8].

References

1. **Porter S.** *The Great Plague* 1st edn. Stroud: Sutton Publishing, 2009, p. 53.
2. http://en.wikipedia.org/wiki/Bills_of_mortality
3. **Porter S.** *The Great Plague* 1st edn. Stroud: Sutton Publishing, 2009, p. 121.
4. http://celticboar.com/texts/plague.pdf, p. 8.
5. http://www.cbwinfo.com/Biological/Pathogens/YP.html
6. http://en.wikipedia.org/wiki/Bubonic_plague
7. http://en.wikipedia.org/wiki/Nathaniel_Hodges
8. http://ids.lib.harvard.edu/ids/view/8282101?s=.25&rotation=0&width=1200&height=1200&x=-1&y=-1

Source: *Occupational Medicine*, Volume 62, Issue 4, 4 June 2012, Page 304, https://doi.org/10.1093/occmed/kqs026. Copyright © The Author 2012.

Reprinted by permission of Oxford University Press on behalf of the Society of Occupational Medicine.

The adjudicator

David Walker

I sing in a choir. Sixty mature males, some technically sound, many not. Formed in a public house 15 years ago following an overture to a retired opera singer by a Friday night regular who thought he could sing. While the maestro got it going, it needed a committee. Good men in tune with the detail and in harmony with the bank manager. But the maestro eventually stretched beyond what was feasible and affordable and the resulting dissonance was intolerable.

His replacement more than filled his shoes. An experienced lady with a musical stave for a backbone. Change through consent. Improvement through pleasure and fellowship. Then one day someone wondered how good the choir was. What were the ways to measure progress?

Invitations were still coming in, though we rarely had a full house. Not a popular choir in the sense of a regular following. A rock band has thousands of fans and they cannot wait to hear the same songs over and over again. In contrast, you hope a male voice choir will sing something different, something you know perhaps. Even singing the same thing differently would be a welcome change.

We entered a competition once under the maestro, came last and had no wish to repeat the experience. So we employed an adjudicator instead.

He was well known and respected around the town. A popular conductor with his own choir and a regular adjudicator at competitions. He sat in for one rehearsal and returned 2 weeks later to deliver judgement. A panning. The acid test was singing quietly, which the choir could not. And singing normally was too harsh. He delivered bad news skilfully by smiling and chuckling with each broadside.

He then turned into a trainer. He sang everyone's notes and demonstrated how he did it with a series of exercises which we copied. He was mustard keen and we lapped him up and his banter.

'You're flat tenors, see if you can ruin this?'

'Are you joining in this time basses? Try and keep up.'

'That was quite nice baritones. Now sing it.'

For his finale, he told us we were quite capable of making a good sound. I left the rehearsal with a sore mouth, chest pain and a buzzing somewhere behind my nose. I had discovered palate and tongue shapes and cranial cavities I did not know I had.

We have had other voice coaches. Good in their way but not followed by sustained change as few of us took personal responsibility to maintain improvement or develop skills further. 'And why should we?' asked a fellow baritone. 'It's a hobby after all. Not easy to learn new stuff when you are knocking on. What if we can't keep up, will we be asked to leave? Will real singers be drafted in? What about auditions, mandatory lessons, competitions, reviews in The Telegraph? There's no telling where it might go.'

Sticking to what you are good at or improving it, learning new stuff, measuring, coaching, testing. Everybody is doing it.

Source: *Occupational Medicine*, Volume 59, Issue 5, August 2009, Page 362, https://doi.org/10.1093/occmed/kqp063. Copyright © The Author 2009.

Stones

Anthony Seaton

How evocative stones are! Each weekend I walk with my grandchildren past a huge smooth boulder and notice the marks on it, made as it was deposited by the melting ice 10,000 years ago. And recently, tidying my study, I came across a piece of oil shale. I live in west Edinburgh, within a couple of miles of the West Lothian oil shale deposits that were discovered by James Young, a chemist, in the early 19th century and became the source of the first mineral oil industry, giving rise inter alia to the word petroleum, oil from rock. But this was not a local stone; it would have confused a mineralogist as it was one I had picked up in a shale mine in the Rocky Mountains in the 1980s, one from my collection of bits and pieces acquired as possibly useful aids to teaching. During the oil crisis of that era, the USA was investigating the use of shale as a source of oil and I had taken the opportunity to research the industry's health effects. All occupational physicians know the story of shale oil cancers.

Here are some of my other memory stones. A piece of haematite, picked up in a local outcrop when I lived in South Wales. Iron was of course one of the resources that allowed Britain to lead the Industrial Revolution and haematite mining continued into the 20th century. A. J. Cronin, before he gave up medicine to become a full-time writer, described haematite miners' lung, a red pigmented form of silicosis. This haematite was of course one reason that the Romans colonized Britain.

A shiny piece of anthracite, found in a run-down coal mine in Pennsylvania; coal was the resource that powered the Industrial Revolution and anthracite was the most sought after type because of its high-energy yield; unhappily, it also proved to be the most dangerous in terms of pulmonary effects on the miners. Coal from Pennsylvania and West Virginia fuelled the Carnegie steel empire and ultimately funded many altruistic works, though the people of those mining areas remained impoverished.

A piece of quartz containing copper ore, from an ancient mine working on Bradda in the Isle of Man. Copper was mined there in the Bronze Age and also sought after by the Romans. It again became economically important in the era when Britain ruled the waves in its copper-bottomed ships. Now it is once more a valuable commodity for cables and electronics, as thieves and scrap metal merchants know.

Finally, a piece of limestone picked up by one of my children on a beach at Sully Hospital near Cardiff. He asked his primary school teacher if it contained an ichthyosaur jawbone, and she was about to toss it aside when she noticed that it did. Yes, stones tell tales, each one shaped by the history of our planet and formed, like us, from the products of the big bang. We have only to enquire of them.

Source: *Occupational Medicine*, Volume 62, Issue 2, March 2012, Page 104, https://doi.org/10.1093/occmed/kqr209. Copyright © The Author 2012.

Why I became a part time occupational physician …

Peter Verow

It could not happen to me! Well it did. Over a period of 2 years, I lost my enthusiasm for work and play. I could hardly sleep yet struggled to get out of bed, dreading the thought of going to work but determined not to give in to feelings of despair. Once I got to work, I went through the motions and isolated myself. My wife was amazed that no one at work commented on my steadily changing state.

Depression affects one in four of us, so why should I have been so adamant that depression could not affect me? I believed it was a temporary state of unhappiness and that I would be strong enough to sort out these feelings. I certainly did not feel I needed the help of other doctors, psychologists or medication. My wife persuaded me that I had to seek help and I made arrangements to see a GP who tried a variety of treatment options but without success. I had thoughts of suicide and eventually I contacted a psychiatrist I knew who proved to be a great support and importantly for my wife who was unable to see any end to my suffering. He provided open access and a rational approach to treatment. We discussed CBT but it was not readily available and we both felt it may not have been right for me at that time. I was also reluctant for yet another person to go through my life's events.

My GP had already advised me that I should take a couple of weeks off sick; however, I felt guilty at doing this and I was certain that 2 weeks would not be sufficient for things to change. I imagined how I could 'legitimately' take sick leave—perhaps break a leg or have something physical that clearly demonstrated that I could not work? I did develop some medical symptoms that required investigation and some mildly abnormal biochemistry results that made me hope I had a 'real' illness and not a psychological one! Not surprisingly, it was the other way around. Perhaps, I should have discussed my fitness to work with an OHP—was I safe to be working when so ill—but which OHP would you go and see yourself?

I continued to feel lousy and recognized that I could not carry on at work. I still did not wish to take sick leave and was fortunate to be able to take a 6 month unpaid sabbatical. The break did not cure my problem but gave me time to reflect and more time for the antidepressants to work. Importantly, I realized I had to make changes in my life.

I returned to work full time knowing that I would either be finding another job or going part time. I discussed this with my HR director who was very supportive. Eventually, I started to improve and the permanent black cloud that had been over my head for so long began to lift. I could even manage to laugh again. I now consider myself back to normal and have learned a great deal from the experience that will certainly influence how I manage others in a similar situation.

We all recognize that patients should not make decisions when depressed, however, such decisions might be part of the answer—the skill for the OHP is finding out how and when you can assist the patient to make them. When depressed, the worst feeling is the 'not knowing' when it will all end. This makes it extremely difficult for the patient to want to talk about their symptoms and the future. Feeling guilty about taking sick leave is exacerbated by the uncertainty of the duration of the symptoms. Do not underestimate the ability of some people (particularly medical) to hide their symptoms. Recognize the psychological impact on individuals who suddenly have to stop or reduce high levels of aerobic exercise (as I did). Likewise, promote the benefits that arise if they can commence such programmes. Doctors should be treated the same as any other individual; however, they frequently have additional difficulties in accessing appropriate care. The partner of the patient is likely to require a great deal of support in these circumstances.

Since admitting to my recent problems, many other doctors have confidentially advised me that they have had similar experiences but were not willing to speak about them openly because of the perceived stigma. I suspect that these perceptions will not change very rapidly; however, I would hope that experiences such as mine may help to raise more openness and discussion of such problems.

Source: *Occupational Medicine*, Volume 59, Issue 8, December 2009, Page 569, https://doi.org/10.1093/occmed/kqp138. Copyright © The Author 2009.

A multidisciplinary clinic for occupational disease

Dorothy Linn Holness

The diagnosis and management of occupational diseases is complex and ideally requires expertise from several disciplines. There is little in the literature regarding clinical models for occupational disease practice aside from the German model for occupational skin disease. The Occupational Disease Specialty Program (ODSP) at St Michael's Hospital in Toronto, Canada, is a clinic dedicated to occupational disease.

The Ontario Workplace Safety and Insurance Board (WSIB) originally operated specialized clinics for workers with complex occupational injuries. In the 1990s, a review suggested the assessment and management of complex cases would be better served at academic hospitals where the worker would receive expert care and clinical education and research activities could be facilitated. This led to the development of the WSIB Specialty Clinic programme with the first speciality clinics focused on injuries starting in 1999. There is a contractual agreement between the WSIB and the hospital and referral to the clinics is by the WSIB. In the early 2000s, it was decided to establish a clinic focused on occupational diseases.

The ODSP was established in 2002. The goals of the ODSP are to provide services related to diagnosis, recommendations for treatment, determination of level of impairment and work restrictions. These are accomplished with a multidisciplinary team and integrated into teaching and research programmes. There are four clinical streams: skin, respiratory, hand–arm vibration syndrome and toxicology. Physician staffing is by occupational medicine specialists and subspecialists relevant to the stream (e.g. respirologist (respiratory physician), allergist, dermatologists). The programme includes support for specialized testing such as patch testing with workplace materials and specific inhalation challenge testing.

The ODSP has an occupational hygienist who assists both with the initial assessment by taking a detailed exposure history and gathering further exposure information as needed. In 2006, a formal return to work (RTW) component was added. This is led by a RTW coordinator, an occupational therapist, experienced in RTW for workers with work-related injuries. The RTW process is a collaborative one involving the RTW coordinator, the occupational hygienist and the physician. Communication amongst team members is facilitated as all are in the clinic together. In working together, the clinicians develop a better understanding of the others' particular skills and all acknowledge the benefit of the multidisciplinary team. The RTW coordinator serves as the main contact with the WSIB, the worker and the employer in the RTW process, thus streamlining and simplifying communication, a critical element in the RTW process.

The ODSP not only provides clinical service to the worker and assists the WSIB in dealing with complex claims but also provides excellent teaching and research opportunities. In addition to occupational medicine trainees, trainees in dermatology, respirology, allergy and clinical immunology and physiatry (rehabilitation medicine) rotate through the clinic, learning about occupational disease in their particular specialty and also the specialized testing. In addition, occupational hygiene and rehabilitation science students have work and research placements in the clinic. The ODSP also provides an excellent opportunity for clinical research.

Source: *Occupational Medicine*, Volume 65, Issue 2, March 2015, Page 106, https://doi.org/10.1093/occmed/kqu149. Copyright © The Author 2015.

Fifty years ago: 'The teaching of occupational medicine to undergraduate medical students'

Anon

A memorandum prepared by the Education Panel and approved by Council for submission to the General Medical Council.

Occupational medicine is the practice of clinical, scientific and other skills in preventive medicine with reference to occupation and the working environment. Since the latter is the environment in which most people spend a large part of their time, all students should be taught to appreciate the importance of its possible effects on the health of those at work.

Occupation is of significance to the practice of medicine in several ways. The nature of a man's work may be wholly or partly responsible for his illness, and to arrive at a correct diagnosis promptly, the doctor must be aware of these possibilities. More commonly the patient's work is important in the management of his illness; the economic and social disturbance of time off work, the need for complete rehabilitation in the shortest period, the possibility or desirability of return to a former job, and consideration of suitable alternative work where there is some residual disability, should be constantly in the doctor's mind. Furthermore, a doctor, whether engaged in public health practice or not, should appreciate the influence of occupation on the health and well-being of a community.

Some of the skills of occupational medicine are common to medicine as a whole and the undergraduate will not require special training within the occupational setting; for example, the treatment of accidents, which is a part of occupational medicine, will be included in the general training of students. Much of the extra knowledge required by occupational medical officers, such as the recognition of dangerous environments and the management and prevention of diseases caused by them, is properly provided by postgraduate teaching. The undergraduate period of training should not be used to train embryo industrial medical officers any more than other types of specialist.

The following recommendations are made for the teaching of occupational medicine to undergraduate students:

1. Ideally there should be frequent reference to the occupational aspects of disease in all clinical teaching.

2. Since it is too casual an approach to the teaching of a subject to leave it to occasional references by different departments, a positive attempt must be made to inculcate in the student an understanding of the significance of the patient's environment.

3. Properly organized works visits are valuable to students in demonstrating the conditions of work in selected industries, emphasizing some of the occupational hazards and showing the special type of medical organization required in industry.

4. An additional means of teaching the subject is through the medium of the socio-medical case conferences which are conducted in hospitals by many departments of social and preventive medicine, in conjunction with the consultant staff.

In summary, the aim of these activities should not be instruction in occupational medicine as such, and the subject must not be presented so that it is an extra dissociated from the rest of the undergraduate course. The teaching must clearly be a part of the general education of students in the role of environment in the causation and management of ill health.

Source: *Occupational Medicine*, Volume 65, Issue 6, August 2015, Page 443, https://doi.org/10.1093/occmed/kqv029. Copyright © The Author 2015.

Originally from: *Trans Ass Industr Med Offrs* (1965) 15, 103. Available at: *Occup Med (Lond)* 1965;15: 103–104. DOI:10.1093/occmed/15.1.103.

Why I became an occupational physician ...

William R. Jenkinson

I had always been interested in work and how to avoid it, so with the value of hindsight a career in occupational medicine was not that unlikely. The decision to pursue a career in occupational medicine came during my early postgraduate days. I can remember as an undergraduate being taught to ask the patient about their occupation, but had no other exposure to the specialty.

Without any clear game plan other than to get as far away from the war zone that was Belfast in the early 80s, I drifted towards general practice. I still believed that a career in general practice would be great, but as I finished my GP trainee year in 1985, I began to doubt that it was really for me. Job offers from Saudi Arabia and Canada quickly followed and as I contemplated them I was unexpectedly offered a partnership in the best practice in my local town. If I did not like it here I reasoned I would not like it anywhere.

Within the first year as a GP partner, I realized I had definitely chosen the wrong career. The nature of the work plus the lack of support wore me down. The practice I joined had traditionally provided occupational health services to many of the local employers. Twice a week I performed a GP clinic in a branch surgery in the grounds of the Moygashel factory for the family and workers of the linen mill. Increasingly I undertook the occupational health work in the practice and found that I enjoyed it, though my level of competence was low.

In 1987 I undertook the distance learning course through Manchester University. This set me on a course of full-time work in occupational medicine, and in 1989, I joined the Post Office occupational health team. I count it a privilege to have worked under Dr Richard Welch who was chief medical officer at the time and Dr Steve Searle his deputy. Both men taught me much. I stayed with the Post Office for five enjoyable years before going to Bombardier Aerospace.

The question is why did I become an occupational physician? I think I can sum that up in two words, interest and opportunity. My interest grew while in general practice and fortunately the opportunity presented itself. Dr Richard Welch stands out as the individual who was most influential in my development as an occupational physician. He gave me an opportunity to work in a highly professional OH unit while I was still very much at the incompetently incompetent end of the spectrum.

I have worked full-time in occupational medicine since 1989 and have enjoyed every day of it. I have had the privilege to ask thousands of employees, 'what do you do?' and to greet the answer with more insight as each year passes. Not many careers can be as fulfilling and varied as occupational medicine.

Source: *Occupational Medicine*, Volume 60, Issue 3, May 2010, Page 210, https://doi.org/10.1093/occmed/kqp192 Copyright © The Author 2010.

Jaw ache—an occupational hazard?

John Storrs

Temporomandibular joint (TMJ) dysfunction is extremely common. The main features are discomfort or pain on opening the mouth and chewing. There may be associated clicking of the joint. The symptoms are commonly unilateral. The causes of TMJ dysfunction are numerous but are often dentally related. An asymmetric bite resulting in jaw ache can stem from a single tooth abscess, dental malocclusion or even unilateral sinusitis. Habitual chewers of chewing gum are obvious candidates for TMJ pain. Stress, in the widest sense, often underlies the painful symptoms. Nocturnal bruxism can be so prominent that the grinding of one's teeth in one's sleep can wake up a partner and in chronic cases causes wear of the occlusal surfaces of molar teeth. Sufferers often think that their symptoms stem from the ear and therefore seek advice from their doctor rather than their dentist. As a result, the patient may be referred to an ENT surgeon or even a neurologist. Eventually, however, TMJ sufferers will find their way to a dentist and it is one of the most common problems that ends up in the outpatient department of a maxillo-facial surgeon.

During my career as a consultant maxillo-facial surgeon, I recall two particularly interesting cases of TMJ dysfunction where understanding the patient's occupation was key to finding a cause and a cure. The first was a secretary who had the usual symptoms of TMJ dysfunction. Careful questioning about her work revealed that she often answered her telephone and continued typing whilst anchoring her phone between her ear and her neck. Problem solved.

The second case was unique for me in over 30 years of clinical practice as a specialist. The patient was a wealthy local farmer. He was middle aged and well adjusted. He had severe pain in his right TMJ. All the usual causes were excluded. After much head scratching, I asked him to give me a detailed account of his daily routine. It transpired that although he had numerous employees, he loved going out on his tractor to work the land. Whilst doing so, he habitually sucked on his pipe which he clenched between his teeth on the left side. I suggested that he should clench his pipe on the opposite side on alternate days. That cured his TMJ pain.

As Ramazzini said, 'When a doctor arrives to attend some patient of the working class ... let him condescend to sit down ... if not on a gilded chair ... on a three-legged stool ... He should question the patient carefully ... So says Hippocrates in his work *Affections*. I may venture to add one more question: What occupation does he follow?' It is true, even in the world of maxillo-facial surgery!

Source: *Occupational Medicine*, Volume 65, Issue 2, March 2015, Page 134, https://doi.org/10.1093/occmed/kqu185. Copyright © The Author 2015.

What clinicians should look for in health and lifestyle apps

Nerys Williams

Smartphones, tablet computers and websites are widely used by clinicians to support patient care and are used by patients to inform, help themselves and challenge their caregivers. Key to the use of this new technology are 'apps'.

An 'app' is simply an application which is downloaded by a user to a mobile device. They can be used for diagnosis, staging or treatment or to help fitness or nutrition and their range is huge. The number of apps available for download from the major players, Google Play (Android) and Apple's App store has exploded over the last 10 years with Apple reporting its 140 billionth download by September 2016 [1]. Statistics for July 2017 show that the most popular apps on the Apple platform are games (making up around 25%) followed by business and education apps with lifestyle making up 8%, health and fitness 3% and medical topics 2% [2].

The Royal College of Physicians (RCP) of London has produced guidance on the use of apps [3] and recommends that clinicians use professional judgement before relying on any information from them. Apps that are used as medical devices should have European CE marking which assures the user that the app meets essential criteria, it works and it should be clinically safe. The RCP likens it to the assurance given by an 'MOT' on a car. The app does not need to be linked to a patient's record for it to need CE marking – any app which uses patient-specific information is considered a medical app and a medical device under the Medical Devices Directives and Regulations and therefore needs a CE mark. Apps which just act as a booking tool for appointments or requests or are revision devices e.g. for the Diploma in Occupational Medicine, do not require a CE mark. Just because an app can be downloaded free of charge does not mean that an app does not need a CE mark – it is its use in relation to patients and patient data which determines if the mark is required. The RCP recommends that users test apps they are planning to rely on even if they do have the CE mark. They suggest running the app in flight mode without wi-fi and seeing how it copes. Testing whether the app clears the previous patient's information is also a useful clinical safety test as some apps keep the previous patient's data and so the potential for input errors arises.

Apps give us the promise of improved healthcare but they should be used with caution and care. Any occupational health professional thinking of developing an app should visit the Medicines and Healthcare Products Regulatory Agency (MHRA) website for information on how to obtain CE marking [4].

References

1. https://www.statista.com/statistics/263794/number-of-downloads-from-the-apple-app-store (3 August 2017, date last accessed).
2. https://www.statista.com/statistics/270291/popular-categories-in-the-app-store/ (3 August 2017, date last accessed).
3. https://www.rcplondon.ac.uk/guidelines-policy/using-apps-clinical-practice-guidance (3 August 2017, date last accessed).
4. https://www.gov.uk/topic/medicines-medical-devices-blood/medical-devices-regulation-safety (3 August 2017, date last accessed).

Source: *Occupational Medicine*, Volume 67, Issue 9, December 2017, Page 721, https://doi.org/10.1093/occmed/kqx134. Copyright © The Author(s) 2017.

Mellifluous

John Hobson

Mellifluous or pleasingly smooth or musical to hear. From the late 15th century and the late Latin, mellifluus from *mel* 'honey' and *fluere* to flow'. Synonyms: sweet-sounding, sweet-toned, dulcet, honeyed, mellow, soft, liquid, soothing, rich, smooth, harmonious, tuneful, musical.

He had the most wonderful speaking voice I have ever heard. If ever a voice deserved the term mellifluous it was his, but it was also authoritative without being autocratic, knowledgeable without being condescending. It was a voice you could believe in. I could hear it in my mind clearly even though I had not actually heard it for many years. I first heard it as a teenager and it played an important part in my choosing science and so medicine rather than art. To me he was the voice of science as well as 'the first invisible star of television'.

Paul Vaughan, who died in November 2014, was the voice of Horizon and Kaleidoscope. He was an Oxford wartime graduate, self-taught orchestral clarinettist and author of award winning books. After a job with a pharmaceutical company, he joined the British Medical Association (BMA) as their youngest staff member despite not having a science degree and became their press officer. His recollections of the BMA were published as Exciting Times. He was also the voice who told us 'The future's bright, the future's Orange'.

I wanted to hear his voice again and followed a link to the BBC archive. Serendipity perhaps or maybe just the space time continuum linking everything together as it likes to do but I found myself watching 'Death of the working classes: Why do the working class in Britain die young?' an episode of Horizon first broadcast in 1988. It presents stark facts about the health risks of lower social class and how of 78 diseases coded by the Office of Population Censuses and Surveys 65 had significant correlations to occupation with only one, malignant melanoma, more frequent in the professional classes. In the documentary there are still shipyards on the Tyne and weaving sheds in Burnley. A young Michael Marmot features and there is an interview with Sir Douglas Black, author of the original Black report in 1980. The Black report demonstrated that although overall health had improved since the introduction of the welfare state, there were widespread health inequalities and that the gap between social class V and I was widening not reducing as was expected. The BBC website notes that 'government statistics released in November 2007 show that this health divide still persists. In 2001–03, men aged 25–64 working in routine occupations (for example, bus drivers, refuse collectors) had a death rate 2.8 times higher than that of men working as large employers or higher managers'. It is sobering to see that despite this knowledge, over thirty years later nothing has changed.

Source: *Occupational Medicine*, Volume 65, Issue 6, August 2015, Page 428, https://doi.org/10.1093/occmed/kqv023. Copyright © The Author 2015.

Why I became an occupational physician …

Ira Madan

Do you enjoy your job? Do you have control over what you do and when you do it? Do you have a good relationship with your colleagues? These are the questions that we frequently ask employees as we know how important these factors are for 'healthy work'.

As a medical student, I enjoyed all aspects of clinical medicine but had no idea what I wanted to do when I 'grew up'. At medical school, a doctor from the Employment Medical Advisory Service gave us an excellent lecture in our public health module. She told us about her work, which was varied and interesting. She stressed the importance of disease prevention and a holistic approach to medicine, phrases hardly ever heard in the rest of my training. The lecture was inspirational and the seed was sown. After doing a general medical rotation, I needed to make a decision. I loved hands-on clinical medicine but still wanted to explore less conventional clinical options, including occupational medicine. I arranged to meet Ching Aw who directed me to David Coggon and Kit Harling. They were welcoming and supportive, had appealing jobs, were well motivated and seemed to enjoy their work. They told me that the scope of occupational medicine was broad; clinical, managerial, National Health Service (NHS), non-NHS, research and teaching—in fact what you make of it. It all seemed a far cry from the cut-throat world of acute clinical medicine, where my consultants moaned about their workload, administrators or the state of the NHS on a daily basis. I was sold. I have since spent 19 years in occupational medicine. I love what I do and my own answer to my opening questions is a resounding 'yes'. I have worked in the NHS, government and academia and have serviced non-NHS contracts. I have worked flexibly in these interesting and worthwhile roles, while bringing up my three children. My colleagues are wonderful and many have become friends. Most importantly, I feel that I have contributed, in a small way, to the health of people at work.

Source: *Occupational Medicine*, Volume 60, Issue 4, June 2010, Page 246, https://doi.org/10.1093/occmed/kqp194. Copyright © The Author 2010.

Reprinted by permission of Oxford University Press on behalf of the Society of Occupational Medicine.

One hundred years of the health and safety laboratory 4

Anon

This controlled explosion (Figure 134.1) was carried out by HSL on the Buxton site as part of the investigation into the Ladbroke Grove rail accident, which occurred on 5th October 1999. The collision occurred at a closing speed of some 230km/hr and resulted in thirty one people losing their lives. An unusual feature of the crash was the major fire which ensued, and HSL's investigation team established that about 6 tonnes of diesel had been explosively released during the accident, when it was atomised and subsequently ignited by the electric power lines. The picture shows a crashworthiness test where a fuel tank was impacted by a vehicle carriage down the impact tract at HSL, and the resultant atomisation of the diesel resulted in a large fireball when it came in contact with an ignition source. Therefore, the likely failure mode of the tanks was demonstrated and related to information obtained from the crash site at the initial impact point of the two locomotives.

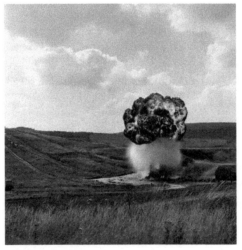

Figure 134.1 Controlled explosion, Buxton
© Crown Copyright 2011.

Source: *Occupational Medicine*, Volume 61, Issue 5, August 2011, Page 340. https://doi.org/10.1093/occmed/kqr113. © Crown copyright 2011.

Slum clinics

Dianne Baxendine

Last year my 16-year-old nephew reminded me of a 7-year-old pact that 'one day' we would visit a developing country for adventure and to serve. So in August 2014, having announced he was now old enough, we set off for India, with 45 others from my local church. Despite volunteering to do anything non-medical, I ended up doing five long, hot clinics in the slums with my brilliant, slightly disparate, holistic team: a local doctor, a nurse, an osteopath, a cognitive behavioural therapist, a pastoral worker and a 14 year old with autism and a flare for overseeing our 'pharmacy'. This consisted of three cardboard boxes containing a mixture of antibiotics, antihelminthics, antiscabitics, vitamins and painkillers all dispensed with a precision to be envied by the NHS. As an occupational physician it was impossible to ignore the many occupational hazards that existed around the slums. Working at height with distinct lack of safe systems was possibly mitigated by the workers' amazing balance. Washing clothes on the ground predisposed women to back, knee and upper limb disorders, but those clothes were clean. There was also exposure to pollution, whole body vibration in the autorickshaws and the risk to life on roads whether from helmetless motorcyclists or avoiding cars, people and animals.

Slum clinics were emotionally challenging and physically draining but uplifting due to the resourcefulness and spirit of the local people. The monsoon season brought flu and upper respiratory tract infections. Where Western health care would prioritize education in self-management, I saw our role as providing symptomatic relief with something as simple as paracetamol, unaffordable to some, whilst truly caring. Physical illnesses were rife, but anxiety and depression often presented as physical symptoms. Our translators were wonderful but addressing such issues required unavailable additional skills and time. I also undertook some interesting workstation risk assessments in a local college but appropriate adjustments would often have required an entirely new office fit. Unusually, my osteopath colleague was on hand to administer treatment—a holistic service indeed.

Questions remain. What is the value of one consultation, without diagnostic facilities and limited communication? Is giving a one-month course of iron tablets a benefit? What about drug side effects? Do the clinics encourage dependence on high-level doctor input, when the priority is improved public health with simple, regular, preventative health care and education, delivered by local trained people?

Would I return? Yes, especially as the local doctor plans to set up more enduring and appropriate health care provision, working with the local church, if funding allows. I believe the experience had more impact on me than any impact I had. The engagement I now have with that community will foster continuing support and relationship. Despite ridiculously different ways and standards of living, I found people are the same, with pride in their families and homes and a strong sense of community. I was privileged to meet them and contribute in a small way to their lives.

Source: *Occupational Medicine*, Volume 65, Issue 3, April 2015, Page 201, https://doi.org/10.1093/occmed/kqu201. Copyright © The Author 2015.

Reprinted by permission of Oxford University Press on behalf of the Society of Occupational Medicine.

Fifty years ago: 'Laser hazards'

John Rich

In 1958 A. L. Shawlow and C. H. Townes postulated the laser. T. H. Maiman succeeded in obtaining laser action in 1960. Before long, lasers are expected to appear in most laboratories and many factories, so it is an opportune time to examine their hazards.

So far lasers have been devised to operate in about 15 frequencies of visible light and in ultra-violet and infra-red modes. It is not surprising that the laser has stimulated an enormous amount of scientific interest with the challenging possibilities of its properties. So many uses were originally proposed that it was dubbed 'a solution in search of a problem'. For the purposes of this paper it will be sufficient to note that uses have been suggested in communications, navigation, cutting and welding, machine alignment, surveying, measurement, rangefinding, photography, military, optical, physical, chemical, biological and medical applications. It is probable that all laser beam properties have significance in biology and medicine. Its optical properties make it easy to direct a small beam at portions of tissue down to microscopic size. When it is focused and its energy is concentrated into a small area, its destructive power may be selectively let loose on structures which absorb light at the wavelength used. Micro-dissection may thus be achieved and there are surgical possibilities.

Though the skin acts as a light barrier, the eye forms not only a transparent window for deeper structures but also a focusing device. Solon, Aronson and Gould (1961) early drew attention to the eye hazards and gave formulae for calculating retinal energy density from a laser beam. They showed that the pulse from a small ruby laser gave a density at least six times that known to cause solar retinal burns, and considered this might be utilized in ophthalmology.

It is known that 6943 A light is practically unabsorbed in the eye until it reaches the retina. It is also of low visual luminosity, and this, with the short duration of the pulse (0-0008sec), makes it scarcely perceived by the patient. So it is possible that an accidental exposure in a laser operator would not be perceived by the victim. Thus, though the laser may be used very successfully for retinal surgery, the laser beam presents a definite hazard to the eye, which, if minimal, can easily be insidious. For this reason it is advisable for laser users, especially in research work, to undergo regular ophthalmic examinations. There should be a pre-employment examination to obtain a norm. Probably only one-eyed or virtually one-eyed workers should be excluded from laser work. Further examinations should be at regular intervals, say six months as an arbitrary period, or whenever an operator believes he has had a beam exposure or develops eye symptoms. Each examination should include visual acuity, visual fields, ophthalmoscopy and slit lamp examination. They will have the three-fold effect of detecting retinal lesions, lesions in other eye structures, such as corneal cataract from unrecognized infra-red lasing, and checking on lax or insufficient safety precautions.

It has been suggested in an occasional survey in the *Lancet* (1964) that the definition of the biological effects of the laser beam raises a problem as great as that originally presented by the discovery of ionizing radiation. Certainly the biological effects of laser light are largely unknown at present, especially in the long term.

Source: *Occupational Medicine*, Volume 65, Issue 7, October 2015, Page 577, https://doi.org/10.1093/occmed/kqv035. Copyright © The Author 2015.

Originally from: Laser Hazards. *Trans Ass Industr Med Offrs* (1965) 15, 147. Available at: *Occup Med (Lond)* 1965: 15;147–149.

A sovereign remedy to all diseases

Anthony Seaton

The title refers to tobacco, from Burton's *Anatomy of Melancholy*. However, I think I know a better one. I was a medical registrar in Stoke-on-Trent, and had just admitted him with haematemesis. He had worked in the pottery industry. I asked the routine question: 'Have you taken any aspirins?' 'Yes, I take one every day.' This was 1964 and people didn't take aspirins to prevent heart attacks then, so I asked him why. 'To keep out the dust' he said.

In that era aspirin was widely used as an antipyretic and analgesic. To medical registrars it was something of a nuisance as not only did it irritate the stomach and lead to bleeding but also, being in all bathroom cupboards, it was a popular drug for attempted suicide. So I advised him that he should avoid it in future and wondered about the reasons for the local folklore that it could prevent silicosis. Stoke was of course the centre of the pottery trade; silicosis had at one time been commonplace from the use of calcined flint in the slip of earthenware and as a bedding material for firing china, though the substitution of alumina in the latter role and attention to occupational hygiene had much reduced its incidence by the 1960s. Perhaps this fall in risk, which started in the late 1940s at the peak of the popularity of aspirin as a home remedy, had reinforced local belief in its efficacy.

While I was giving this sensible advice, John Vane was studying the mechanisms of action of aspirin and the prostaglandins, work that led to his Nobel Prize in 1982. Some hints were soon to arise that aspirin's anticoagulant properties might be of benefit after myocardial infarction and from the late 1980s the drug has been used routinely in this situation. Now we hear that it may also have preventive actions with respect to cancer, especially adenocarcinomas, and possibly even have a role in cancer treatment.

Medical textbooks of the mid-19th century mention many treatments for fever, including mercury, lead, tartar emetic and even, extraordinarily, flagellation. Graves comments in his textbook that he had been informed that poor people, who couldn't afford a doctor, were more likely to survive fever than the rich. No wonder! It must have been a relief to many that the synthesis of aspirin in Bayer's laboratories in the 1890s allowed physicians to deploy a much less toxic remedy, one that became so popular that it could be used with impunity to prevent even silicosis. As I have watched the evolution of the understanding and uses of this remarkable molecule and its anti-inflammatory properties, I wonder what biological advantages willow trees get from making salicylic acid and, intriguingly, whether the potters of Stoke-on-Trent knew something we didn't.

Source: *Occupational Medicine*, Volume 62, Issue 5, 5 July 2012, Page 365, https://doi.org/10.1093/occmed/kqs067. Copyright © The Author 2012.

Why I became an occupational physician …

Henry N. Goodall

Two decades ago, many occupational physicians came from general practice, having spent 5–20 years as general practitioners (GPs). I started as assistant to an established GP with a busy varied urban practice in Bournemouth, 12 home visits a day and one-in-three nights and weekends. Six months later, my senior partner had a coronary; I very quickly learned how not to do general practice, on my own, which is not in the books. Moving to Southampton as a GP in 1974, I added half a day per week of Accident & Emergency work. When our senior partner left, I inherited his multiple varied part time occupational health (OH) commitments.

Ten years later, I began to realise that I wasn't doing the OH work as well as I would like and, separately, that I could no longer practice medicine to the standard to which I had been trained, in National Health Service (NHS) general practice, which was then being suffocated by stagnant bureaucracy and poor morale. I was only able to 'scratch the surface' of people's lives, as a GP, and wanted to make more of a difference. I could see the future of the NHS and knew that it would take 10–15 years to happen. Several GP colleagues had fallen victim to illness, due to overwork. I decided that I wanted to live beyond the age of 50 years.

I enrolled in the Manchester Distance Learning Course, with Ewan Macdonald as my tutor, and a year later was offered an opportunity to join Ford Motor Company, by Monty Brill, as a full-time trainee, two immense strokes of good fortune, to be guided by such icons, from the start. My lasting memory of the Manchester residential weeks was of the dry uncomfortable windowless lecture room, which experience taught me more about relative humidity, ergonomics, occupational psychology and the design of the working environment than many hours of study.

Ford of Britain then encompassed almost every working environment. Being embedded in a large multi-national company exposes an occupational physician to management, trade union and commercial pressures unknown in the NHS, which demand the highest standards of judgement and communication; there is no hiding place on the shop floor. Following early retirement, after 15 years, I moved from corporate to consultancy work, also teaching younger colleagues in specialist training, more good fortune. Three years later, another move to Atos Healthcare, not only with the challenges of wholly paperless (and secretary-less!) working and extensive daily travelling but also increased professional isolation.

Having to reinvent your career is essential to continued success (and employment!). Throughout, the SOM has provided contact with enthusiastic supportive colleagues, high-quality CPD and genuine friendship. You consistently meet kinder, friendlier and more humble colleagues in OH, than elsewhere in medicine. Making 'more of a difference' to UK plc has been a privilege, throughout that time. Looking back, I wish that the opportunity had come 5 years earlier, but life rarely gives you the opportunity and the facility together. Two decades on, it is good to know that I made the right call.

Source: *Occupational Medicine*, Volume 61, Issue 3, May 2011, Page 156, https://doi.org/10.1093/occmed/kqr014. Copyright © The Author 2011.

Fashion victims campaign: responses from clothing retailers

Paul Grime

A recent filler article in this journal [1] signposted a campaign for justice for Bangladeshi garment workers [2]. In December 2013, I emailed 13 clothing retailers asking five questions about their commitment to good working conditions for garment workers. Seven retailers replied, all by email; two with links to relevant sections on their websites and five with bespoke responses. None answered the five questions systematically or completely. The following is a brief summary of the responses received:

1. Does your company import clothing made in Bangladesh or other developing countries?

   Two retailers said that they sourced products from Bangladesh. Two said that they worked with supplier factories in many countries, developing and developed, but not including Bangladesh. One said that their product care labels indicate their source.

2. Do you set minimum workplace standards for your suppliers?

   One retailer required factories to provide decent working conditions and the right to join a union, and described a range of other benefits. Three described measures they take to improve workers' conditions, including human resource management, crèche facilities, professional skills training, building stronger communities, reducing poverty and enforcing codes of conduct for workers' rights. Two also required adherence to standards of the Ethical Trading Initiative (ETI) [3]. One required industry benchmark standards to be met if they were higher than national legal standards.

3. Do you ensure they pay their workers a fair wage?

   Two retailers said that they required their supplier factories to pay at least the legal minimum wage, and both were committed to the principle of a "Living Wage" that covers basic needs with some discretionary income.

4. Does your company support the international Accord on Fire and Building Safety?

   Two said they did.

5. What assessments have you made recently of your supply chain to ensure significant and sustained improvements in the working conditions of garment workers?

   Six retailers described in various levels of detail what they required of their suppliers and how they assessed compliance. These included adherence to ethical principles and audits, root cause analyses and action plans on non-discrimination, forced labour, child labour, wages and hours, working conditions, health and safety, environment and freedom of association. They also described other ways that they work with suppliers to improve workers' lives, including factory visits, workshops and conferences, updating suppliers on current local ethical issues, workforce investment, managing homeworking and raising money for children's scholarships. One retailer said that ensuring good labour standards throughout their supply chain was not only the right thing to do, but also made good business sense.

I was unable to find answers to any of the questions on the websites of the retailers that did not respond. The responses sound encouraging, but if we are to eliminate injustice on the scale represented by the collapse of the garment factory building in Bangladesh in 2013, there is clearly much still to do.

References

1. **Grime P.** Fashion victims. *Occup Med (Lond)* 2014;**64**:66. Google Scholar Crossref PubMed
2. *New Justice for Bangladesh.* http://www.methodist.org.uk/mission/world-church/asia-pacific/bangladesh/new-justice-for-bangladesh (1 February 2014, date last accessed).
3. Ethical Trading. *Initiative: Respect for Workers Worldwide.* http://www.ethicaltrade.org (1 February 2014, date last accessed).

Source: *Occupational Medicine*, Volume 65, Issue 4, June 2015, Page 316, https://doi.org/10.1093/occmed/kqv003. Copyright © The Author 2015.

Reprinted by permission of Oxford University Press on behalf of the Society of Occupational Medicine.

What's in a name?

Mike Gibson

Some time ago, I sat as a medical member on a tribunal appeal where the appellant (patient) had been refused employment and support allowance (ESA). On his claim form, completed by his mother, he was stated to have ADHD and Tourette syndrome. We did not have too much confidence in the medical assessment carried out after his initial application, particularly as the examining health professional (or was it Microsoft's spell checker?) reported that he was suffering from 'turrets'. But where does the name Tourette's come from? The eponymous medical syndrome is now abbreviated to Tourette syndrome but it used to be called Gilles de la Tourette syndrome. Names with particules such as de la, de or d' can be abbreviated to the geographic name, for instance 'd'Estaing' as in the case of the former French president whose full name is actually Valéry Marie René Georges Giscard d'Estaing. Georges Albert Édouard Brutus Gilles de la Tourette (1857–1904) was born in St Gervais les Trois Clochers, near the city of Loudun and nowhere near La Tourette which is a small village in the south east of France, not far from Lyon. The name Gilles de la Tourette indicates a link to a particular estate or an aspiration to be thought of as having noble origins. The modern usage of Tourette is therefore grammatically incorrect—a bit like calling a disease after the place of discovery rather than the eponymous discoverer. In France, the condition is known as SGT (Syndrome Gilles de la Tourette). Tourette started his medical studies in 1873 at Poitiers but then moved to Paris where he studied under and later worked for the eminent neurologist Charcot. Tourette described the symptoms of his syndrome in nine patients in 1885, using the name 'maladie des tics' [1]. Charcot renamed the condition 'Gilles de la Tourette's illness'. In 1893, a disgruntled former patient shot Tourette in the head. Although he recovered, he began to experience mood swings and in 1902, his worsening mental state caused him to be dismissed from his post. Gilles de la Tourette died on 26 May 1904 in a psychiatric hospital in Lausanne but his name lives on. And what of our appellant with Tourette's? He had been expelled from school, college and work experience because of his violent behaviour, tics and coprolalia. It did not take too long to decide the appeal in his favour as he was virtually unemployable.

Reference

1. **Gilles de la Tourette G.** Étude sur une affection nerveuse caractérisée par de l'incoordination mortice et accompagnée d'écholalie et de coprolalie. *Arch Neurol* 1885;9:19–42 (158–200).

Source: *Occupational Medicine*, Volume 65, Issue 5, July 2015, Page 397, https://doi.org/10.1093/occmed/kqu123. Copyright © The Author 2015.

Tales of Kieran: The occupational physician's odyssey 7—Aromatherapy

J.A. Hunter

It is quite remarkable what an academic appointment can do for one's career. Ever since Kieran became occupational physician at Linbridge University, it has been hard to pick up a medical journal without seeing his name, or more disturbing, his picture peering out from the pages of some of the more tabloid publications. At first, it was the odd book review and then letter to the editor, as he tried out his new-found respectability. Then he progressed to writing opinion articles in some of the more esoteric periodicals, before I noticed his name appearing in adverts for conferences for this, that and the other. These are the types of conference that always take place in London, have an opening address by a member of parliament or media celebrity who never turns up, and the 'expert' speakers know next to nothing about the subject they are speaking about. [The only part of the body that Kieran has any experience of repetitive strain in is the temporo-mandibular joint.] Most alarming are the conference fees they ask for, most of which would humble the salary of most hospital managers. Yet there seems to be a never-ending stream of the things in the post, so presumably somebody must go to them.

It all came to a head when in the same week Kieran had written to the editor of one British medical journal, had the book that he had edited reviewed in an American journal, and in another British medical journal had written one of the leading articles. This was heavyweight respectability on a large scale, even though I didn't understand what the hell he was writing about.

Unable to deny Kieran his moment of glory, I paid him a visit, usually a good way to get a free lunch in his college if he was in a good mood. It was strange, therefore, to find Kieran in a most despondent state, and rather than the journals left conspicuously around and open at the relevant pages, Kieran was studying the job section intently.

'What on earth is the matter?! Surely your career is what you've always wanted?' I exclaimed, as Kieran asked what I thought of community paediatrics in Ghana.

'The job was fine', Kieran finally explained, 'until the University Chief Executive went on one of these stupid health conferences for managers. You know, the ones that are always in London, cost a fortune and have an opening address by a member of parliament who never turns up.' I nodded knowingly. 'Well she has got this idea into her head that the Occupational Health Department should be offering benefits to the University's workforce as befits a major employer.'

'Well there's nothing wrong with checking a few blood pressures or cholesterol is there?' I offered, as Kieran's nostrils began to flare.

'Blood pressure! Cholesterol!' Kieran bellowed. 'The crazy woman wants me to arrange on-site aromatherapy and reflexology, not to mention post-traumatic stress counselling, chiropractic and acupuncture. If she thinks that I'm spending my time tickling feet and sticking perfume up people's noses, she can find another occupational physician.'

And that was that. I didn't get lunch. I didn't see Kieran's job advertised either, even though I kept a close eye on the job sections for a good few months. It was only when I came across a paper describing an outbreak of occupational dermatitis in health care staff exposed to aromatherapy agents that I was able to reassure myself that all was well at Linbridge. I do wonder whether they are tickling feet, mind you.

Source: *Occupational Medicine*, Volume 53, Issue 4, June 2003, Page 297, https://doi.org/10.1093/occmed/kqg059. Copyright © Society of Occupational Medicine.

Why I became a respiratory physician with an occupational interest

David Fishwick

My grandfather was born in St Abb's head lighthouse at the turn of the previous century. He worked for the Northern Lights Company and lived an interesting and highly uncertain life, moving from lighthouse to lighthouse with a young family in tow. One of his tales stuck in my mind from childhood, and involved a lighthouse keeper, off shore on a rock station, cleaning the varnish off an old wooden floor using petrol, as part of routine maintenance. The ensuing inferno almost wiped out the station, and its three keepers were only saved by a passing ship. Even as a little boy, I thought to myself, 'work can be dangerous!'

During my training in Manchester, I seemed drawn by respiratory medicine, but it was my experience at Wythenshawe Hospital that sealed my fate. Not only did I become passionate about helping patients with breathing problems but I was also given the opportunity to enter the world of research. Manchester has always been a great industrial city, and after SHO jobs, Tony Pickering offered me a research role involving this heritage. Had I known at the outset that I would talk to >3000 cotton workers, day and night, about their breathing and work exposures, maybe I would have displayed slightly less enthusiasm to take part!

For the first time in my life, I witnessed workplaces that could be unpleasant, noisy, dusty, hot and humid, and it dawned on me that these types of conditions, certainly globally, were probably commonplace and certainly very different from my personal experience of work.

Tony was inspirational as a supervisor and highly knowledgeable about workplaces. He pushed me to take the Associate of the Faculty of Occupational Medicine exam and to this day, I do not regret the extra time and effort required to do this. This experience formed my professional life as a dedicated respiratory physician with an interest in occupational disease. I now work as a consultant respiratory physician in the National Health Service and as the chief medical officer at the Health and Safety Laboratory. I am reminded daily that there is a substantial body of work yet to be achieved in order to render workplaces less risky in terms of their ability to harm the lungs. This work has to be achieved in the shorter and longer term by a mix of disciplines, so that the outputs are sensible, simple and practically useful. My contribution to this process, I believe, is by dealing with workers with occupational diseases but having a firm grounding in all things occupational.

As for the future? Well, business as usual for me perhaps, but we all miss a trick if we do not allow doctors, when training, to mix a specialty interest such as respiratory medicine with occupational training. I am convinced that this type of approach will populate our country with a unique resource to continue to deal with and assess workers developing the traditional occupational diseases.

Yes, work can be dangerous, but good work is vital to all our futures.

Source: *Occupational Medicine*, Volume 61, Issue 5, August 2011, Page 320, https://doi.org/10.1093/occmed/kqr051. © Crown copyright 2011.

Reprinted by permission of Oxford University Press on behalf of the Society of Occupational Medicine.

An unusual occupation with novel hazards

Paul Williams

In my capacity as his general practitioner I knew him relatively well. The majority of healthy middle-aged men in regular employment never go anywhere near their GP over the course of many years so he was a little unusual in his attendance pattern. He also had a tendency to present with unusual work-related health problems. On this occasion, he presented with marital problems that had arisen as a consequence of his last work-related health problem. He was a bit fed up and wanted someone to sound off to and I guess that was my role in his life, particularly as he knew I was bound by a professional oath of confidentiality. 'All those years I've supported my family and no complaints.' I settled in for the time it would take for him to finish presenting his complaint suspecting it would be a bit longer than the average two and a half minutes. 'No complaints when I was out all night, coming home early to get the kids their breakfast. No complaints when I took them to school so she could head off to work. No complaints when I came home and did the shopping, cleaning and so on. No complaints when we were one of the few families to have new appliances and nice holidays. No complaints when I'd pick the kids up and get the tea after the shortest of naps before heading out for another night's graft.' The problem had been triggered by his need to stay awake to do his work as well as being somewhat of a model new man. 'No, all those years of amphetamines to keep me awake and no complaints. But just once it messed with my mind a bit and now she won't speak to me! It's not fair!' His habitual use of amphetamines had provoked morbid delusional jealousy some months beforehand. I finally persuaded him of the need for psychiatric intervention and he was now well on the road to recovery. His wife on the other hand wasn't being quite so conciliatory about the negative impact this episode had brought to their relationship.

The other work-related condition I had seen him for had been some years beforehand. He had developed a shoulder problem and when I ascertained that his work was at factory premises and involved manual handling and awkward posture of the upper limb, the embryonic occupational physician within me had pricked his ears up. Of course I asked him his occupation. 'I'm an industrial burglar' he said matter-of-factly. 'Never touch domestic dwellings, mostly night shift work, with some physical lifting and carrying and use of crow bars.' And of course incarceration had been an issue at times, but that's a different kind of occupational hazard.

Source: *Occupational Medicine*, Volume 65, Issue 5, July 2015, Page 379, https://doi.org/10.1093/occmed/kqu205. Copyright © The Author 2015.

Fifty years ago: 'Emery Pneumoconiosis'

A.O. Bech, M.D. Kipling, and W.E. Zundel

Emery is a rock that occurs in Naxos, Turkey and the United States. The composition of the rock varies somewhat, but approximately it is 50 per cent corundum (aluminium oxide), 30 per cent haematite or magnetite and the remainder complex aluminium salts.

In the past emery was the abrasive in bonded grinding wheels, but it is now only used as an abrasive powder applied to a bob or mop, incorporated on a belt or in a wax preparation. For rough grinding a bonded wheel is used, for finer grinding the emery is glued to a bob of leather or wood with a leather or cloth covering, for scutching and polishing the emery is glued to a mop made of calico, linen or cotton and for fine polishing emery flour is incorporated in a bar of wax or fatty material with which the mop is dressed. The presence of excessive dust in the atmosphere of some polishing shops has been given as a cause of difficulty in recruitment of polishers (Weill, 1950). Enough dust may be produced in polishing large objects to require several changes of face-masks during the working day. Burkart (1960) estimated that one belt polishing machine, using 150 mesh powder, gives off 90 G of respirable dust in a week, representing the 1–2 per cent of particles from the abrasive and metal that were under 5µ. Polishing is still something of an art, though in some workshops traditional techniques are replaced by automatic polishing machines, and emery to some extent, for polishing, by synthetic corundum.

Confusion may arise in the investigation of the health of grinders and polishers because the term grinder may apply to a fettler of castings, who is exposed to foundry sand, because sandstone grinding wheels are still in use for certain trades as in the manufacture of garden tools and because the word emery is often used for the other abrasives, natural corundum, synthetic corundum and carborundum (silicon carbide) as well as for the natural product. In emery polishing there may be exposure to the dust of natural emery, natural or synthetic corundum, to glue and the fabric of the mop, together with metal from the material under treatment.

Since we saw abnormal radiographs in an emery polisher in 1959, we have endeavoured to ascertain the extent of the risk of this work by a survey of thirty-four workers in two polishing shops, by obtaining information from other chest physicians in the region and by inquiry from doctors in industry. As a result of this inquiry we have been able to investigate four metal polishers with abnormal radiographs who were under the care of other chest physicians, and two who were found to be abnormal at pre-employment examinations. In one polishing shop two out of thirteen workers showed radiological abnormalities and in the other, one out of twenty-one. None of these polishers gave a history of exposure to dust other than that occurring in metal polishing.

We found that prolonged exposure to the dust is necessary before radiological changes develop; the average for our ten cases was thirty-seven years and the incidence of changes was not high. Of the thirty-four polishers from two factories, radiological changes were apparent in five.

Source: *Occupational Medicine*, Volume 65, Issue 8, November 2015, Page 606, https://doi.org/10.1093/occmed/kqv036. Copyright © The Author 2015.

Originally from: Emery pneumoconiosis. *Trans Ass Industr Med Offrs* (1965) 15, 110. Available at: *Occup Med (Lond)* 1965;15:110–115.

Piles

John Hobson

It was the most untidy office I had ever seen. On every available horizontal surface including the floor, chairs and window sills, there were piles of documents and manuscripts, theses, books and journals. He was a senior academic and I was there to discuss the analysis of a research project. I heard him invite me in but couldn't see him until he stood up from behind a paper barricade he had built at the front of his desk. He ushered me over to a table whose surface had long since disappeared and cleared a pile of papers from a chair. At random he dumped it on another pile on the floor. At one point during our meeting, somewhere hidden, a stack of papers collapsed the heard but unseen falling tree in the forest. Without noticing he continued talking p numbers and statistical tests but I was preoccupied with the state of the place. How did anything ever get found or done? How much of it had been read let alone marked? There could be buried work of genius here from students who had long since qualified and who never knew what became of their work. I was so struck by the place that I lost focus on what he was explaining. Not surprisingly the research never got analysed. How could a statistician, someone who makes sense of complex situations and produces clarity from chaos ever choose to exist in such a mad written material maze?

A few years ago a national stationery retailer carried out a survey of office tidiness. They estimated there were 449 million pieces of wasted paper on the UK's desks which if piled high would reach the height of The Shard 148 times. Over a quarter of the 2000 people surveyed said they had received complaints from their managers and work colleagues about the state of their desk and nearly half admitted to losing important paperwork because their desk was so unorganized. Dr Chamorro, a professor of Business Psychology at UCL said: 'A messy desk can have a very serious impact on our stress levels and therefore our happiness in general. Over half of our respondents said that their stress levels increased purely at the sight of their messy desk. Our participants' wellbeing could be significantly boosted by simply devoting a bit more effort and resource to keeping their office environments tidy and well-organised.' Others have written of the stress from having piles of unread medical journals although these days my piles tend to be electronic and relate to unread emails something that can feel like a never ending computer game with the impossible objective of a clear inbox. One study did find positive correlations between self-reported tidiness, life satisfaction and subjective happiness so perhaps untidiness at work is a stressor and occupational health should be involved? The last word however belongs to Albert Einstein: 'If a cluttered desk is a sign of a cluttered mind, of what, then, is an empty desk a sign?'

Source: *Occupational Medicine*, Volume 66, Issue 5, July 2016, Page 357, https://doi.org/10.1093/occmed/kqv025. Copyright © The Author 2016.

Why I became an occupational physician …

Giuliano Franco

In the early 1960s, I moved from my home town of Trieste in north-eastern Italy, to the renowned University of Pavia, where as a third-year medical student, I chose to attend the Institute of Occupational Medicine in preference to the crowded wards of the medical departments. It was a choice that influenced my future. In those years, the institute, chaired by Professor Salvatore Maugeri, included clinical sections, outpatient services, laboratories, a toxicology section and other facilities. The social, stimulating and demanding environment allowed students to combine hard and effective work with easy and efficient learning and develop strong ties with residents and doctors. After my degree in medicine and a 2-year period of military service, Professor Maugeri made me an offer that I could not refuse: to undertake an academic career working as his assistant. His outstanding management abilities coupled with exceptional empathy resulted in the foundation of the prestigious Institute of Research and Care, which was later named after him.

In the 1970s, I worked in the cardiology section studying the cardiovascular effects of carbon disulfide, in the clinics of occupational medicine developing skills to diagnose occupational disorders and in the toxicology laboratory studying the effects of metals and solvents. After completing specializations in cardiology, internal medicine and occupational medicine in the early 1980s, I was appointed as an associate professor of occupational medicine.

In the early 1990s, I was appointed chair of occupational medicine at the University of Modena. Even though the name of Modena is inextricably associated with that of Bernardino Ramazzini, the founder of occupational medicine who taught there at the end of the seventeenth century, at the time of my appointment, there was no academic occupational medicine facility. That period was exceptionally challenging, stimulating and engaging. I developed growing international relationships fostered by active participation in associations such as European Association of Schools of Occupational Medicine, Union Européenne des Médecins Spécialistes (European Union of Medical Specialists) and International Commission on Occupational Health. Meanwhile, thanks to the incorporation of Directive 89/391 into Italian law, I had the opportunity to develop a professional activity in the university and the teaching hospital and to improve the formative process of the school of occupational medicine through the implementation of a quality system. At that time, I assumed that some mandatory interventions, performed by doctors, were either obsolete, useless for the effective protection of workers' health or could be carried out by nurses or simply omitted. This observation led me to apply the principles of scientific evidence, not without resistance from colleagues, to the daily activities of occupational physicians, a journey still to be completed.

It might be observed that I never made a demanding career choice and I came into occupational medicine by luck, coincidence or serendipity? An answer can be found in a reflection by Cesare Musatti, the founder of psychoanalysis in Italy. He said that whoever began an academic career did so because they did not want to stop being a student but wanted to delay the traumatic entry into a new environment.

Source: *Occupational Medicine*, Volume 61, Issue 8, December 2011, Page 589, https://doi.org/10.1093/occmed/kqr147. Copyright © The Author 2011.

Philosophical Transactions: 350 years of publishing at the Royal Society

Eva Baranyiová

Carlton House Terrace, London. A prominent address in the heart of the buoyant city, yet a quiet and dignified house when one enters. It has been the residence of the Royal Society of London since November 1967, the fifth residence since 1660, when the Society came into existence.

The conference was one of the 2015 events to celebrate the beginnings of scientific publishing in England: *Philosophical Transactions of the Royal Society* was the name of the journal, a well-known and respected science forum to this day. Its first issue appeared on March 6 of 1665 (two months later than the French *Journal des Sçavans*) (Figure 147.1).

The conference of historians was a tribute to Henry Oldenburg who, a native of a German Bremen theological family, came to England, and became the Secretary of the Royal Society (1662–1677), after extensive travels around scientific Europe. Although he was not a scientist himself, his education, diligence and talents (he spoke German, French, Latin, Italian and English) made him an ideal personality to make and keep vivid contacts with scientists in England, France, Holland, Germany and elsewhere. The beginning of the Enlightenment era saw an eruption of discoveries, disputes and criticisms among scientists, and Oldenburg became the spirit of communication among them. He knew how to extract and summarize the information from their letters. He published abstracts, notes and comments on experiments, book reviews, in the newly established

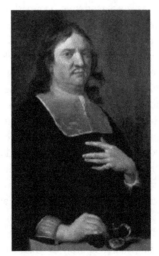

Figure 147.1 Heinrich (Henry) Oldenburg, the Society's first Joint Secretary and mastermind behind the Philosophical Transactions.

Reproduced with permission from Baranyiová E. (2015). The scientific journal: past and present. *European Science Editing*. **41**(2):30. http://www.ease.org.uk/wp-content/uploads/ese_may15.pdf

journal to which he was commissioned by the Royal Society. His enthusiasm led him to finance the 136 issues he published until his death in 1677 although it was licensed by the Royal Society.

Of course, not only Oldenburg, but the entire period since early days and various aspects of science publishing, were the themes of two plenary and twelve parallel sessions. There were also two evening public events (The experience of scientific publishing, and The future of scientific publishing) dealing with more present themes, such as the changing forms of peer review, possible loss of data due to e-publishing, quality of papers, history of collecting reprints and their value, order of authors that should be set before the work begins. In the second one, training of young authors was stressed and the role of editors herein. The present style prose of papers was questioned in the internet era – do we need all that text? And the impact factor was discussed too, not liked by authors and editors.

The Royal Society also published special theme issues, Philosophical Transactions A, physical sciences papers, and Philosophical Transactions B, life sciences papers. Both issues deal with scientific questions of early days viewed from today's perspective, all written by well-known scientists in the respective fields. One can find most interesting commentaries on works published by Newton (1672), by Caroline Herschel (1787), by Lister (1673), Faraday (1832), Joule (1850), Maxwell (1865), and by others who made important contributions to science. Another 17 articles on personalities in biological sciences beginning with Leeuwenhoek (1677) "Concerning little animals" appeared in the series B.

Scientific publishing has been changing at an ever increasing pace. We should learn how to adapt the peer review that will remain an important quality guarding tool, and look for more efficient ways of communication in science in the 21st century, possibly even moving away from the scientific publishing of today. We are not yet fully aware of the potential offered by using the web in this endeavour.

Source: *Occupational Medicine*, Volume 65, Issue 9, December 2015, Page 738, https://doi.org/10.1093/occmed/kqv188. Copyright © The Author 2015.

Reprinted with permission from Baranyiová E. (2015). The scientific journal: past and present. *European Science Editing*. 41(2):30.

Occupational histories

Mike Gibson

Despite the exhortations of Ramazinni in the 17th century to ask all patients about their occupation, many general practitioners do not record a patient's occupation in their notes. The occupational physician appreciates that such knowledge is essential when advising on a patient's fitness for work and even more so when determining if a condition is work related. A key part of the occupational medicine curriculum is the importance of the occupational history and one of the requirements in the long case for the MFOM clinical examination is to obtain a work history. Sometimes, obtaining an accurate work history from patients is like drawing teeth. Memory can be inaccurate and sections forgotten, 'mis-remembered' or deliberately withheld.

There is, however, an accurate way of obtaining an occupational history but not in this country. Thirty years ago, I was working at RAF Hospital Wegberg, near Mönchengladbach. As Officer Commanding Medical Wing (quaintly called the Registrar of the Hospital), I was the general practitioner for the hospital staff but I was also in charge of all the support staff, including the typing pool, who were German. One day in 1985, I had to officiate at the retirement ceremony for a delightful lady who was one of the typists. I therefore called for her work record so that I could prepare my speech.

This was the first time I had had the opportunity to view an official German work record (Arbeitsbuch). As you may expect, it was comprehensive and logical, detailing the date of starting each employment, the job title, the date of leaving and, helpfully, the individual's explanation of the reason for leaving. This particular lady had started work at the age of 18 in a confectioner's shop in 1937. One year later, she had moved to a chemist's shop. The column in the record labelled 'Reason for Change' recorded that she had moved 'Besser zu mich selbst'—to better myself. One year later, she moved again, this time to work for the Abwehr—a military intelligence organization—to train as a typist. Again the reason for changing jobs was to better herself. In 1946, she was engaged to work for the British Army of Occupation (later the British Army on the Rhine—BAOR) and thence to the Royal Air Force. But this time, the reason for leaving was honest, simple and incontrovertible. It stated merely, 'Den Krieg verloren' or 'Lost the War'.

You can imagine that such a work record would be helpful to general practitioners, occupational physicians and epidemiologists. It would also be useful for compensation claims where this relates to historical exposures such as for mesothelioma, bladder cancer and hearing loss. However, experience in the UK suggests that such logic and organization may not be achievable.

Source: *Occupational Medicine*, Volume 65, Issue 7, October 2015, Page 516, https://doi.org/10.1093/occmed/kqv045. Copyright © The Author 2015.

Risk assessments: Good and bad

Anthony Seaton

Many years ago, I had the responsibility once a month of doing a tuberculosis clinic in deepest West Virginia. The small town that I drove to was the site of the State penitentiary—it was said the citizens had been polled on whether they wished to have this or the State university and had opted for the gaol in the belief it would provide more jobs. On one occasion, a small and inoffensive-looking patient was led in, handcuffed on both wrists to burly warders. I ensured that he was taking his drugs and making satisfactory progress and arranged to see him again the next month.

After he left, curious to know why the security had been so apparently excessive, I asked the nurse, a local woman, what he was in for. She told me that he had been done for armed robbery. The story was that he had lived in the town all his life and was known to most in the community. One day he had walked in to his local bank, pulled out a pistol and demanded of the cashier that he hand over all the money. The cashier, recognizing that death from acute lead poisoning was an occupational hazard of bank employees, wisely complied but took the sensible step of calling the police when the robber left, giving them his name and address which, as he was also a customer, was known to the bank. The police went round to his house where he was found counting the money on his kitchen table. He received a severe sentence, an occupational hazard of robbers.

Hazards, foreseeable adverse consequences of an activity, are quantified as risks in our Control of Substances Hazardous to Health (COSHH) assessments. The risk of being a victim of an armed robbery is low for any individual, even in Appalachia, but the outcome may be fatal and is always traumatic. The cashier clearly made a snap-risk assessment and decided on a wise course of action. The risk of being apprehended after performing an armed robbery on one's own bank in one's own community must be high, even in Appalachia. My poor patient must have been unfamiliar with the practical importance of risk assessment and learnt that failure to make one could lead to serious consequences. A lesson to us all.

Source: *Occupational Medicine*, Volume 62, Issue 7, October 2012, Page 540, https://doi.org/10.1093/occmed/kqs110. Copyright © The Author 2012.

Why I became an occupational physician ...

John Aldridge

National Service in 1953 took me first to the Royal Armoured Corps at Bovington with a variety of units, a large REME workshop and a busy medical centre. I took the opportunity to drive a Centurion tank. A Short Service commission took me to the Cambridge Hospital in Aldershot as a trainee medical specialist and later to the Queen Alexandra Hospital in Millbank. About to marry a QARANC nursing sister I succumbed to the financial inducement of a permanent commission.

Attending the advanced medicine course at the London Hospital I first encountered Dr Donald Hunter, an enthusiastic teacher who always emphasized the importance of the occupational history in relation to the illness. I subsequently acquired MRCP in Edinburgh, taking Tropical Medicine—well taught at Millbank—as a special subject, and was posted as medical specialist to the Military Hospital in Tripoli, Libya, responsible for general medicine and paediatrics. Returning after 3 years to the Military Hospital at Chester I decided to return to civilian life necessitating a probable change of specialty. Fortuitously, while in Cheshire, I met Pat Barry of Associated Octel and Mike Flindt of Unilever who introduced me to Industrial Medicine.

Appointed to the Reed Paper Group under Gordon Smith I obtained DIH in company with Peter Taylor who I had known as a student and also in the Middle East; Peter was the RAF medical specialist in Cyprus who reviewed the fitness to fly of patients of mine requiring air evacuation to the UK. We remained close friends until his untimely death.

At Reeds, I became interested in what seemed the relatively neglected area of occupational mental health and when in 1963 IBM sought a doctor interested in 'stress', I was fortunate to be appointed. I remained there for 24 years until my retirement and witnessed the rapid advances of data processing in diminishing packages.

To broaden my education and understanding of mental ill health, I did a part-time clinical assistantship for Dr Roger Tredgold, a consultant psychiatrist at UCH with a special interest in mental health at work and I also became a co-therapist in a therapeutic group. I took part in other group activities organized by the Tavistock Institute and others and saw the introduction of group dynamics as a management development tool. Not always successful!

In the late 1960s I assembled a small group of senior occupational doctors to discuss mental health at work and this grew to a more structured occupational mental health discussion group [1]. Interest in this aspect of employment expanded until the more general recognition of its importance. With colleagues we also organized several international meetings with the emphasis on the mental health of the organization and its employees.

I was privileged to play satisfying roles with the Royal Navy, the Society both centrally and locally, and the Faculty becoming Dean in 1986.

Reference

1. **Fingret A.** Occupational mental health: a brief history. *Occup Med (Lond)* 2000;**50**:289–293.

Source: *Occupational Medicine*, Volume 62, Issue 5, 5 July 2012, Page 336, https://doi.org/10.1093/occmed/kqs066. Copyright © The Author 2012.

PTSD induced by the trauma of subordinates: The Robert Gates syndrome

Eric Altschuler

In July of 2011, Robert Gates resigned as US Secretary of Defense after serving in that position for 4½ years under two Presidents of different political parties. In the Author's Note to his recently published memoir *Duty* (Vintage, New York, 2014), Gates explains his surprising choice to resign as Defense Secretary, 'Toward the end of my time in office, I could barely speak to them [soldiers] or about them without being overcome with emotion. Early in my fifth year, I came to believe my determination to protect them …was clouding my judgment and diminishing my usefulness to the president …' In the book, Gates notes that 'the hardest part of being secretary for me was visiting the wounded in hospitals … and it got harder each time'. In reflecting on the penultimate page of the book Gates writes, '… in my mind's eye I could see them [injured soldiers] lying awake, alone, in the hours before dawn, confronting their pain and their broken dreams and shattered lives. I would wake in the night, think back to a wounded soldier or Marine I had seen … and in my imagination, I would put myself in his hospital room and I would hold him to my chest, to comfort him … so my answer to the young soldier's question … about what kept me awake at night: he did'.

That is, Gates has ongoing and longstanding recurrent recollections, dreams and awakenings about the injuries of soldiers under his command. These were so significant as to force him to retire from his job. If these recollections were about trauma he himself had experienced, Gates would meet criteria for post-traumatic stress disorder (PTSD). As best is known, Gates personally did not experience such trauma, so his feelings and emotions are solely induced by trauma sustained by his subordinates. Loved ones or caregivers for patients who have undergone trauma can experience PTSD symptoms [1]. But this situation is different because PTSD is being experienced by the person who ordered the traumatized individuals into the situation that induced the trauma. PTSD induced by trauma of subordinates likely occurred to others in the past either in the pure form as here or a mixed form induced also by personally experienced trauma and is likely an important workplace hazard for civilian and military war commanders.

Reference

1. **Clawson AH, Jurbergs N, Lindwall J, Phipps S.** Concordance of parent proxy report and child self-report of posttraumatic stress in children with cancer and healthy children: influence of parental posttraumatic stress. *Psychooncology* 2013;**22**:2593–2600.

Source: *Occupational Medicine*, Volume 66, Issue 3, April 2016, Page 182, https://doi.org/10.1093/occmed/kqv201. Copyright © The Author 2016.

Fifty years ago: 'Problems of a group occupational health service in Lancashire'

F.H. Tyrer

Rochdale lies on the extreme north-eastern fringe of the Manchester conurbation, flanked to the north and east by the bleak Pennine moorlands which separate it from the West Riding of Yorkshire. Its population has declined over the last thirty years, and at the 1961 census was 85,785 compared with 88,429 in 1951. Cotton manufacture, both spinning and weaving, was the predominant local industry during the nineteenth century, and although the town has shared in the general shrinkage of this industry, it remains an important one. Only three firms have more than 1000 employees. Man-made fibres are increasingly being used, together with cotton, in weaving, and a recent development is the coating of fabrics with P.V.C. and similar plastics.

The six member firms had a geographical distribution covering most of the points of the compass within a radius of three miles of the town centre, and preliminary reconnaissance showed very quickly that local industry generally was of similar distribution. It was stressed to all member firms that whether or not they were large enough for this to be a statutory requirement, their first line of defence in emergency should be one or more employees trained in first-aid. Our experience has confirmed the findings of other group services that treatment is the first thing expected by employers and workers from an occupational health service. This establishes a bridgehead in the winning of confidence, after which gradually preventive work can be developed and extended. Requests from managements for examinations specifically related to fitness for jobs, and for advice on environmental problems have steadily increased. Byssinosis in cotton card rooms is probably the major industrial hazard of the area. Virtually the only work done on this problem has been that of Professor Schilling and others working under his direction; but what has hitherto been almost entirely lacking in the cotton spinning industry is a health protection service which by continued supervision of card room workers and advice at the appropriate time could prevent permanent disablement.

In all parts of the country absence after injury or long-term sickness tends to be unnecessarily prolonged simply by lack of communication between those responsible for the patient's treatment, on the one hand, and those responsible for his resettlement in suitable work on the other. The occasional individual whose injury or illness has been so severe that it seems obvious he will require resettlement through the official machinery may be referred to the D. R. O. [Disablement Resettlement Officer] but the vast majority tend to continue off work so long as they are attending out-patients, if not specifically told they are fit to resume.

Few employers take the decision to join purely as a result of intellectual conviction; emotional attitudes, for or against, seem to me to be much stronger factors. Genuine altruism is not so rare as cynics believe; and 'keeping up with the Joneses' and brushes with the Factory Inspector may also play a part. So, too, may personal experience of hospitals through past misfortunes of directors or members of their families. Man is not nearly so rational a being as he likes to pretend—and payment for an occupational health service is certainly not the only form of expenditure which can be governed by the heart rather than the head, as the advertising industry understands full well.

Source: *Occupational Medicine*, Volume 65, Issue 9, December 2015, Page 703, https://doi.org/10.1093/occmed/kqv037. Copyright © The Author 2015.

Originally from: Problems of a group occupational health service in Lancashire. *Trans Ass Industr Med Offrs* (1965) 15, 132. Available at: *Occup Med (Lond)* 1965;**15**:132–139. DOI: 10.1093/occmed/15.1.132.

Working in the shadow of a thin blue broken line

John Challenor

A recent paper on protracted sickness absence in police officers by Summerfield [1] and a synchronous commentary by Wessely [2] has brought back memories of my own role as a police medical advisor. The move from a richly varied portfolio of industrial and commercial occupational health (OH) was calculated and very carefully considered. In my late 50s, it would most probably be my last career shift before I reached the then statutory retirement age of 65.

Two eminent professors of OH looked at me sternly when I mentioned my plans. One expressed concern and muttered something about dens and lions and the other said, 'I wouldn't do that if I were you'. But my nature and addictiveness to challenge swept aside these and many other expressions of concern and I was subsequently employed as a police medical advisor between 2001 and 2009.

Summerfield's paper highlights not only a general OH maxim but also a ubiquitous police service phenomenon. 'The medicalisation of non specific symptoms allied to social rewards that create perverse incentives, reliably prolongs disability'. More specifically, 'the definitive role of traumatic stress claims was not to produce a fit officer but to support his wish for ill health retirement and pension' [1]. Wessely's comment was more succinct. 'For police officers, who have not made it to senior command, there comes a point when chasing criminals or grappling with rioting students is no longer for you' [2] although in my experience seniority was not a bar to significant psychosocial symptoms arising in relation to management conflict.

Amongst the cited references in the first paper is Cahill-Canning's MBA thesis [3]. In the section on organizational culture and sick leave Cahill-Canning states, 'the strongest correlation between taking sick leave and organisational cultural factors was with [a] sense of team spirit'. A sense of team spirit and social network predicts reduced sickness absence—a phenomenon that is reflected in Wessely's comments.

Reading these remarks has evoked memories of shared experiences in a police OH unit that were blood spattered, tear stained and often sullied by the spittle of bitterness and irrationality brought by a small but significant proportion of patients who clearly held dear to them that they were deserving of something much more than a salary.

It was a far from perfect system and it was often challenging to remain objective and politically neutral. At times, there was optimism for a tiny number of patients who were positive and incentivized regarding return to work. More dismal memories remain vivid but mellow with the passage of time as the parts we all played in systems within systems become the stuff of reminiscences.

But in my experience and those of colleagues, the views described by Summerfield and Wessely remain a cardinal feature of police OH work. This is unlikely to change under the present circumstances. It's time to get out the ruler and make it a solid blue line.

References

1. **Summerfield D.** Police force blues: reflections on protracted sickness absence. *Br Med J* 2011;**342**:d2127.

2. **Wessely S.** A police officer's lot is not a happy one. *Br Med J* 2011;**342**:d2252.

3. **Cahill-Canning E.** *To what extent is sickness absence in the Metropolitan Police Service influenced by organisational culture and the quality of the employer–employee relationship?* MBA thesis, Greenwich School of Management, 2003.

Source: *Occupational Medicine*, Volume 61, Issue 6, September 2011, Page 382, https://doi.org/10.1093/occmed/kqr094. Copyright © The Author 2011.

Reprinted by permission of Oxford University Press on behalf of the Society of Occupational Medicine.

Why I became an occupational physician …

Jerry Beach

My first contact with occupational health came at medical school in Newcastle. As part of the undergraduate curriculum we all went to visit a workplace. My visit was to Thermal Syndicates Limited, a company manufacturing fused silica and other glass products in Wallsend. I remember walking through vast production areas, climbing over enormous piles of sand, and being intrigued about the process of turning sand into useful products. At the time I thought I was getting a half day away from studying but the fact it remains one of the more memorable parts of my under-graduate years suggests something stuck. I later volunteered to lead a group of students on another workplace visit to the Hayhole Lead works also in Wallsend so my interest in occupational health was obviously piqued by this early exposure.

My next real contact was when working as a junior doctor in South Shields in the 1980s, a place which seemed to be awash with impressive pathology. One of the more notable conditions I remember seeing was mesothelioma, a consequence of the local docks and merchant marine. From there I moved to a job as a registrar in Newcastle upon Tyne, part of which was with David Hendrick in the chest clinic where I learnt about the clinical aspects of occupational lung disease. The cases that stick in my mind most were the investigations of fibrosing alveolitis and hyper-sensitivity pneumonitis. I visited barns and rooted around looking for mouldy hay and I learnt how to take blood from a pigeon and prepare it for an inhalation challenge. I then moved into a research job, also supervised by David Hendrick, looking at asthma and airway responsiveness among shipyard workers and apprentices at the VSEL yard in Barrow in Furness. I was fascinated by the process and the sheer scale of the operation. I took every opportunity I could to get out into the shipyard and look around, including acting as a 'bag man' for the hygienist on the project for a week.

My next move was to the Institute of Occupational Health at Birmingham, to the joint training job with Lucas Industries which allowed me to express the frustrated engineer within trying to get out. Not only would people allow me to go into their workplaces and see how some of the most complex pieces of machinery in the world were built but they actually seemed to enjoy my interest. The university component of the job allowed me to become involved in research and teaching, which I enjoyed, and I got to see some fascinating clinical cases of occupational lung disease in the Birmingham Chest clinic. I was hooked.

In hindsight, I was lucky. I almost stumbled by accident into a job which suits me well. The variety of work and intellectual stimulation continues to keep me enthused. There were decision points when I had to actively select occupational health, but as other contributors to this column have mentioned, serendipity certainly played its part.

Source: *Occupational Medicine*, Volume 62, Issue 6, September 2012, Page 443, https://doi.org/10.1093/occmed/kqs126. Copyright © The Author 2012.

New Stress Check Programme in Japan's workplace

Tomoyuki Kawada

In December 2015, the Japanese government established a legal backing for workers' mental health based on the Stress Check Programme [1]. This programme was instituted by an amendment of the Industrial Safety and Health Law in 2014 and is implemented at least once a year at all workplaces with 50 or more employees. The employers cannot access the results of the Stress Check of any individual employee without the employee's consent and must provide the employee with the opportunity for an industrial physician interview if the employee requests one. In 2005, the Japanese government had already established a legal backing for workers' health based on the number of extra working hours, to prevent cardio- and cerebrovascular diseases. This combination of legal backing for improving the physical and mental health of the employees is expected as a useful health promotion activity in the Japanese workplace.

However, there is no clear academic evidence yet of the usefulness of the legally established mental health programme in preventing suicide or psychiatric illness in Japanese workers. Wada *et al.* conducted a cohort study of the stress response measured by the Brief Job Stress Questionnaire (BJSQ) to identify the onset of depression [2]. Among 1810 participants, 14 developed depression during a mean follow-up period of 1.8 years, and the hazard ratio (HR) (95% confidence interval) in the subjects with a BJSQ score for depression in the highest quartile was 2.96 (1.04–8.42); the adjusted HR showed the same tendency. As the number of events was only 14, it was difficult to obtain a reliable estimate of the risk for mental disorders such as depression after adjusting for several independent variables. I have experience of using the BJSQ in cross-sectional studies but have found no clear evidence of the association between the score on the BJSQ and the risk of work-related mental disorders.

In an attempt to resolve this query, Madan and Williams systematically reviewed the evidence for the effectiveness of pre-employment health questionnaires in predicting health and employment outcomes [3]. Unfortunately, the authors found no papers in the literature addressing mental health outcomes and recommended assessment of the prospective benefit of health screening questionnaires.

In addition, no screening process for high-stress workers or a standard management procedure has been established yet. Nevertheless, each company is expected to allocate a budget and is obliged to provide an annual report to the government. Although the Stress Check Programme is a unique method, industrial physicians have to make efforts to communicate with any highly stressed workers to improve workers' mental health. As there are no reports of experience of using a legally backed Stress Check Programme for workers from other countries, useful information could be obtained on the effectiveness of the new health promotion system established in Japan for improving the mental health of workers.

References

1. **Kawakami N, Tsutsumi A.** The Stress Check Program: a new national policy for monitoring and screening psychosocial stress in the workplace in Japan. *J Occup Health* 2016;58:1–6.
2. **Wada K, Sairenchi T, Haruyama Y, Taneichi H, Ishikawa Y, Muto T.** Relationship between the onset of depression and stress response measured by the Brief Job Stress Questionnaire among Japanese employees: a cohort study. *PLoS One* 2013;8:e56319.
3. **Madan I, Williams S.** Is pre-employment health screening by questionnaire effective? *Occup Med (Lond)* 2012;62:112–116.

Source: *Occupational Medicine*, Volume 66, Issue 7, October 2016, Page 527, https://doi.org/10.1093/occmed/kqw057. Copyright © The Author 2016.

Reprinted by permission of Oxford University Press on behalf of the Society of Occupational Medicine.

Jelly beans and jumbo jets

Anthony Seaton

How many jelly beans can you get into a jumbo jet? This was a question asked at interview of a young graduate seeking employment. His answer, that he really had no idea, may have explained his lack of success. When I read this in the education section of *The Guardian,* my immediate thought was why someone had asked such a strange and apparently unanswerable question. But by now, you will have your answer ready … or perhaps not. If not, here's mine. You can easily get one in and maybe a packet in your pocket. If you are a salesperson for the confectioner, you could probably get a case or two in the hold, but if you wanted to take a lot in your hand luggage, it would be well to check with the airline that the jelly beans would not, being some sort of gel, be regarded as potentially explosive fluids. It turns out to have been a rather interesting question, designed to examine the candidate's ability to think laterally. I really don't know how I would have answered it if asked in my interviews for jobs as a young doctor—maybe I was asked such questions and this explains why at one stage I only got the eighth job I was interviewed for.

It was only a decade later, around 1970, that I read Edward De Bono's book on lateral thinking and realized how important, but how dangerous, this can be in medicine and science. Advances in science come both from incremental change, step-by-step building on what is known and also from radical new ideas. Nowadays, the first of these is usually the product of well-equipped teams of researchers, whereas the latter is dependent upon individuals; papers by lateral thinkers have only one or very few authors, whereas most scientific papers are compiled by teams. Lateral thinkers, like James Lovelock of the Gaia world, are an endangered species as the members of grant committees, editorial committees and most referees tend to be step-by-step people and nervous of endorsing radical new ideas.

I believe that there is a lateral thinker in all of us, a persistence of the innocence of childhood when we asked questions of grown-ups and puzzled over the answers, an innocence that seems to be washed away too easily by the formal and dogmatic education my generation received. In contrast, in art classes one is constantly encouraged to get out of one's comfort zone and one hopes that the current undergraduate medical curriculum fosters a similar attitude. I have practised a trick for keeping the innocence alive. It has been my habit to avoid big medical meetings of like-minded colleagues (save for the purposes of meeting old friends) and to attend meetings on subjects outside my expertise, usually multi-disciplinary. Like a sometimes bewildering television panel show, it gives one the opportunity to make connections and generate new ideas. How many jelly beans? Only connect!

Source: *Occupational Medicine*, Volume 65, Issue 3, 1 April 2015, Page 209, https://doi.org/10.1093/occmed/kqu163. Copyright © The Author 2015.

Society of Occupational Medicine Golden Jubilee Travelling Fellowship 2017

Nerys Williams

Thanks to the SOM Golden Jubilee Travelling Fellowship I was able to attend an advanced education course on physical activity in the workplace held in Reykjavik in October 2017. It was organized by NIVA, an organization founded in 1982 in Helsinki and allied with the Finnish Institute for Occupational Health (FIOH). NIVA has been an active player in the field of occupational health and safety education for 35 years and is now the only institute in Europe that focuses solely on an international and advanced level of occupational education. Course participants largely come from the Nordic countries (75%).

The course, held over 3 days, was unusual for an occupational health course in the diversity of both lecturers and audience. The lead lecturer was a professor with expertise in sports science ably assisted by an epidemiologist, health economist and experts in computer technology. The audience was made up of occupational physicians, physiotherapists and PhD students from sport and exercise medicine.

The course covered published research, mostly originating in Denmark, on the impact of physical activity programmes in workplaces. Examples of slaughterhouse and care workers were used to illustrate outcomes and some of the difficulties in setting up programmes. These difficulties included motivating employers to participate and maintain interest, recruiting staff to avoid bias and the limitations of studies because of unplanned changes in the work being undertaken. The studies favoured the stepped approach to study design where each group of participants went through both 'control' (i.e. no activity) and 'intervention' (activity) stages at different times.

The research presented suggested that if workers undertook a few minutes of resistance exercise each day then they experienced a reduction in musculoskeletal complaints. But the difficulties in getting unmotivated staff to participate were clear. The group discussion identified that in the case of care staff, their willingness to help residents and patients may be the key to getting them to exercise. The experience of those in the room was that training care staff to show residents and patients exercises, including resistance exercises, to do each day could be a way forward given that staff often work in the sector because of their desire to help others and they often put their own health second. The NIVA team supported this view and emphasized the importance of physical activity to their own organization so much that they have placed short training videos using both no equipment and simple cheap elastic thera-bands on their website (https://niva.org/workout-take-a-227-min-break).

The course was an excellent challenge to my current thinking on physical activity in the workplace. This was less about gyms and physical exercise and more about simple activity. The impact of a few minutes resistance training per day in reducing musculoskeletal complaints was convincing but so was the need to avoid prolonged sitting. The course has highlighted that in-activity designed into jobs is the cause of musculoskeletal pain and obesity and has motivated me to look differently at the workplace.

Source: *Occupational Medicine*, Volume 68, Issue 4, June 2018, Page 272, https://doi.org/10.1093/occmed/kqy028. Copyright © The Author(s) 2018.

Shaking all over

John Hobson

As a medical student I remember very clearly a visiting American research doctor who on his first day introduced himself to me by firmly shaking my hand and telling me his name. Strange to think this now but then it was unusual, particularly from more senior doctors, and it left a lasting impression. Over the years my handshaking practice has developed to the point where I always shake hands with my patients, both at the beginning of the consultation and usually at the end. The patient who won't or 'can't' shake hands provides useful clinical information but that is another story.

What does a handshake mean? They are a form of greeting, or parting or seal an agreement. Many years ago in a BMJ personal view, Edwards spoke about contact with patients. He felt that consultations which ended in a handshake indicated that the patient was saying 'Thank you'.

When I had the privilege of working in France, I soon realized it was the land of the handshake. At work, it was obligatory to shake everybody you met by the hand. Working in an open plan office with 46 other people meant that turning up for work could be a major ordeal. Forty-seven people each shaking hands with each other means over 1000 handshakes first thing in the morning or about one person hour. More strange was the fact that it was definitely taboo to shake the same person's hand twice in one day. The French have an impressive ability to remember names and exactly which hands they had already shaken. More than once, miserable English man that I am, I offered a hand to be turned down with the words 'Non, deja vu'.

With time I adopted strategies to cope with all this repetitive upper limb activity. It became extremely time-efficient to arrive in the office as early as possible so that rather than making the rounds of your colleagues, they visited me at my desk.

In the factory the handshaking continued. Workers would spot you from the other side of the building and cross the shop floor simply to say 'Bonjour, ça va?' and shake you by the hand. There were also interesting variants of the practice: the Mechanics or Dirty-hand-handshake consists of shaking the proffered wrist rather than the hand; the Right-hand-occupied-handshake, e.g. on the telephone, involves shaking the upside down left hand; and the Postprandial handshake, which never occurs before lunchtime so they are more certain that you have washed your hands.

Does such frequent epidermal contact spread microbes? After all the French are great kissers as well. Perhaps the exchange of skin flora on a friendly basis helps build immunity? Some of my more squeamish expatriate colleagues believed that the shaking of hands was responsible for the increase in upper respiratory tract infection they experienced when working abroad. However, whatever the loss of productivity and resultant upper limb disorder and minor infection, I have to say I found all that civility rather nice.

Source: *Occupational Medicine*, Volume 66, Issue 9, 19 December 2016, Page 712, https://doi.org/10.1093/occmed/kqw123. Copyright © The Author 2016.

Reprinted by permission of Oxford University Press on behalf of the Society of Occupational Medicine.

Why I became an occupational physician …

Robert Willcox

One year after qualifying in 1972 I was invited to join the staff of a large London church where I worked for 3 years keeping my stethoscope warm in part time General Practice. During that time I founded a Christian professional theatre company which ran for 7 years with a permanent theatre in central London and a touring element performing regularly at the Edinburgh Festival. In returning to medicine, I needed a nine-to-five job in order to continue managing the theatre. Occupational Medicine fitted the bill and although initially boring with routine medicals, a career full of fascination developed. Most companies seem to have been British (Petroleum, Airways and Broadcasting Corporation!)

The patient with the most dangerous job was Al Capone's driver (before reasonable adjustments came in!).

The most intriguing study was hooking up the BBC Symphony Orchestra members with portable ECG's in the Royal Festival Hall and matching the ECG output against the complexity of the score. A significant finding was an ergonomic one that the cellists had a marked tachycardia six bars before the trombones behind them were due to come in! The CMO Dr Ann Fingret introduced me to Steve Williams, the first organizational psychologist to develop a validated stress questionnaire assessment and thus my career-long interest in the psychology of the workplace was born.

The most scary moment was presenting to a paying public audience in Central Hall, Westminster, on workplace aspects of migraine.

I have enjoyed a rich variety of workplaces and some seriously helpful mentors. Belonging to a small speciality, I count myself fortunate to have been working with colleagues and friends who are prepared to pioneer unusual areas combining clinical and business expertise. Tropical disease training with British Airways has led to a global perspective with International SOS developing Occupational Health training in a worldwide context. The group (IAPOS) founded 35 years ago by Dr Stanley Browne, world famous leprologist who drew together Chief Medical Officers of global companies, Mission and NGO doctors and tropical disease specialists, has been a particular stimulation.

The need for people with good medical and managerial skills is as great as ever, particularly if they have the courage to make it fun as well. As a speciality we continue to need those who dare to be different and have the courage of their convictions.

Source: *Occupational Medicine*, Volume 62, Issue 7, October 2012, Page 532, https://doi.org/10.1093/occmed/kqs102. Copyright © The Author 2012.

Preparing for retirement

Stephen Deacon

Retirement for some doctors is defined by their terms of employment and normal retirement age for pension benefit. However, many occupational medical services are now provided by independent doctors often with a portfolio of customers. This situation provides a degree of choice in retirement date with the option of reducing practice commitments as a prelude to full retirement. However, in the final year before retirement, the doctor will need to make important decisions about managing their professional arrangements. In all likelihood there will not be alignment between the different dates for renewals of subscriptions, licensing and revalidation.

Thus, preparations for retirement will likely involve some pragmatic decisions. For instance, it would appear unreasonable to pay significant annual subscriptions only to retire the following month. Also, while revalidation has introduced absolute requirements for maintenance of good medical practice, the evidence base for appraisal is an aggregate accumulated over a year not necessarily in a linear manner. Thus, there may be little need for a final few months' educational activity if the doctor has accumulated a good deal of evidence in the preceding appraisal period and there is no intention to undertake further annual clinical appraisal or seek revalidation.

The financial costs of medical subscriptions, educational activities and medical indemnity insurance to sustain medical practice are significant and may influence decisions about possible part-time working. Good medical practice implies the doctor will continue to participate in active education and reflection until the date of retirement. Sir Keith Pearson in his recent review of revalidation has advised that 'it is important not to lower the evidence requirements or the standard of assurance that revalidation provides to patients'. Thus, a combination of cost and revalidation requirements may be factors that will deter older doctors entering part-time practice as a prelude to full medical retirement. This is an unfortunate 'unintended consequence' of revalidation. Part-time working would be of some assistance to tackle the manpower crisis in our specialty demography. In coming years, there will be a large manpower loss due to the 60% of baby boomer doctors aged over 55 years entering retirement with insufficient replacement trainee numbers.

Ceasing medical practice and revalidation arrangements requires surrendering the licence for medical practice. This is achieved by notifying the GMC. However, the retired doctor may chose to remain on the Medical Register in order to retain their medical title and possibly undertake advisory work using their medical experience but not engaging in actual medical practice. Should the doctor wish to be removed from the Register then the GMC requires references from two recent employers to affirm the good standing of the doctor.

Hence doctors approaching retirement should consider their preparations. Anecdotal discussions with senior peers involved in administering revalidation and clinical appraisals suggest that a degree of flexibility may be observed in educational arrangements during the final year before retirement. However, more formal guidance from the GMC would be helpful to assure a fair and consistent approach to retirement arrangements.

Source: *Occupational Medicine*, Volume 67, Issue 5, July 2017, Page 343, https://doi.org/10.1093/occmed/ kqx070. Copyright © The Author 2017.

Reprinted by permission of Oxford University Press on behalf of the Society of Occupational Medicine.

Fifty years ago: 'The scope of occupational medicine in a university health service'

Anthony Ryle

While university occupational health includes classical, formal environmental health problems such as laboratory safety, radiation and so on, its central concern, I believe, should be with the main function of the University as an institution, namely, teaching and learning. The aim of a University Health Service in this context is to minimize failure and under-achievement among students. To achieve this aim involves an extension of the doctor's role beyond the detection and treatment of illness, and beyond a concern with formal psychiatric illness, to a concern with what I call the 'irrational transaction' between the student and his teacher at the University. To develop a Health Service, which can work along these lines, one must follow certain stages. Firstly, one must create a satisfactory clinical service, because upon this depend the basic attitudes of the students and the University to the doctors. Secondly, the doctors will intervene, on behalf of student patients, with their tutors where illness or disability has interfered with their functioning. Thirdly, partly through such intervention, the doctor can begin to extend the general understanding of his role to include a recognition of the part he can play in understanding the tutor–student interaction. If he is accepted in this role, then a fourth stage becomes possible in which the Health Service is formally involved in policy making, in teaching of tutors and so on. When the doctor in his occupational role is faced with a student who is a psychiatric or an academic casualty, I think he should ask himself two kinds of question. Firstly, he must ask what, in the history and the personality of this student, predisposed to psychological or academic breakdown. Secondly, what in the institution may have promoted, and what could have prevented or may limit his breakdown.

Meanwhile, how much can be done by a University Health Service to modify the institution in such a way as to diminish problems among students? At Sussex, various processes are under way which I think can have such an effect. In the first place all students in severe academic difficulty are reviewed by a central committee of all the Deans on which I sit, and at which medical information on those students who give permission can be presented. In this way, recognition of the role of psychological factors in promoting work difficulty has been established throughout the University. In the case of students with such difficulty who are under treatment, direct discussions with the tutors involved can go some way further towards enabling the tutor to understand what is happening between him and the student, a process which must at times involve him in examining his own reactions. Finally, by seminars and 1-day conferences for tutors, we have undertaken some more or less formal education and exchange with tutors about the irrational components of the teaching situation. I believe that it is in these ways, and in cooperating with others in research into the teaching process, that a University Health Service can carry out its specific form of occupational medicine.

Source: *Occupational Medicine*, Volume 68, Issue 1, January 2018, Page 59, https://doi.org/10.1093/occmed/kqx190. Copyright © The Author(s) 2018.

Originally from: The scope of occupational medicine in a university health service. *Trans Soc Occup Med* (1968) 18, 28–29. Available at: *Occup Med (Lond)* 1968;18:28–29.

A blue patient and exploding factories

Anthony Seaton

In those days it was usual for house physicians and surgeons to cover casualty in the evenings and overnight. For the young doctor it was great experience though whether it was best for the patient might be doubted, but we were keen and we learnt a lot from being thrown in at the deep end. And every so often we came across real rarities.

He walked in, apparently well but concerned that he had turned blue. His wife confirmed that it had occurred that afternoon for no apparent reason and, sure enough, he was quite deeply cyanosed. He wasn't breathless and I could find no abnormalities in his heart or lungs. His only symptom had been a recent sore throat for which he was being treated by his general practitioner. Recently qualified, I had not had time to forget my lectures on haemoglobin, and suspected methaemoglobinaemia. The pathology technician confirmed the diagnosis by spectroscopy of his blood and the scene was set for a major piece of drama in front of the nurses. Drawing up a syringe-full of methylene blue I slowly injected the dark blue liquid intravenously into the dark blue man and, in front of our eyes, he turned pink. I suggested he stopped his sulphonamides and he went home happy.

The editor tells me that these anecdotes must bear some relation to occupational medicine. Well, a decade later in 1973, as a young chest physician I was working in a hospital across the road from a chemical factory. We did not have a casualty department but we did have one emergency role. The factory made polymers using acrylonitrile, C_2H_3CN, otherwise vinyl cyanide, pretty toxic stuff which on burning produces hydrogen cyanide. We were instructed by the factory doctor in the urgent treatment of cyanide poisoning by giving intravenous sodium nitrite, to convert the patient's haemoglobin to methaemoglobin which binds cyanide, followed by sodium thiosulphate. Fortunately it was never necessary but I did decide to write a novel about an explosion and fire at a chemical factory, with a cloud of toxic gas drifting over the local village. Chapter one was nearly finished when, on a weekend in June 1974, a factory in Flixborough making caprolactam for the manufacture of nylon leaked 40 tonnes of cyclohexane which blew up, destroying the factory, killing all the workers present and damaging most of the houses in the nearby village. Two years later, in the Seveso region of Lombardy, a small factory making an intermediate for hexachlorophene, leaked 6 tonnes of vapour, including a kilogram of 2,3,7,8 tetrachlorodibenzodioxin (TCDD), from a reactor into the local community where it killed thousands of a small animals and caused chloracne in several hundred people.

All occupational physicians were able to impress their partners by diagnosing dioxin poisoning in Mr Yushchenko while the media speculated on the cause of his, happily temporary, disfigurement. But, alas, chapter one is as far as I got with my novel, and factories continue to explode.

Source: *Occupational Medicine*, Volume 63, Issue 4, June 2013, Page 280, https://doi.org/10.1093/occmed/kqt018. Copyright © The Author 2013.

Why I became an occupational physician …

Malcolm Gatley

I qualified in 1957 at Liverpool University where I had hardly heard of occupational medicine.

After a year in house officer jobs, I considered a career in ENT and became a senior house officer, but after 18 months, I decided that it was a mistake, although I had no clear idea about the future.

Then I spent 11 years in general practice, part of which was in Halewood near the Ford factory where many of my patients worked. I saw patients with problems attributed to their jobs and others requesting sick notes.

Realizing that I knew nothing of the work of these patients, I visited the Ford factory. I found out that a doctor was employed there but I was not able to meet him.

Then an incident occurred that was to be the turning point in my career. A heavy parcel arrived by post addressed to me in error. In it was Hunter's Diseases of Occupations. It looked interesting, and I kept and read it (after paying). By the time that I had finished it, I knew what I wanted to do.

I knew that there was a university department of occupational health in Manchester headed by Professor Tim Lee. Coincidentally, I was then considering returning to the Manchester area where my family lived. In 1968, I moved back there (still in general practice) and, very shortly after, applied for a vacancy of 'Appointed Factory Doctor'. To my amazement I obtained the post and gradually found other part-time jobs in occupational health.

By 1973, I was spending half my time in the field and wanted to work full time in it. I was then very fortunate to obtain another two part-time posts in the food industry and with the Central Electricity Generating Board. With these I was almost full time in occupational medicine and left general practice.

After 2 years on Professor Lee's fascinating course at Manchester University, I obtained the DIH in 1975. During and after this time, I was very grateful for Tim Lee's help and advice in becoming accredited.

Later, much of my work was in the then 'Cinderella' field of NHS occupational medicine, and I was very attracted by the challenges in that developing branch of the specialty.

The final miracle in my career was in 1983 when I obtained the first consultant post in this region. It combined clinical duties in a district health authority (later trust) with a regional advisory role. Gradually the department grew and provided occupational health care to many outside organizations. I spent a highly interesting and rewarding 15 years until my retirement from the NHS in 1998.

Looking back, I benefited from a series of very fortunate and unexpected coincidences in a career from which I have enjoyed the greatest job satisfaction.

Source: *Occupational Medicine*, Volume 62, Issue 8, December 2012, Page 619, https://doi.org/10.1093/occmed/kqs103. Copyright © The Author 2012.

Reprinted by permission of Oxford University Press on behalf of the Society of Occupational Medicine.

Golden Jubilee Travel Fellowship 2016

Folashade Adenekan

While undertaking higher specialist training in occupational medicine in the UK, I developed a particular interest in the management of psychological ill-health in the workplace, probably as a result of this constituting three quarters of my workload. I attended a talk on the management of 'sick doctors' in the UK by the Practitioner Health Programme (PHP) and was intrigued by the support and resources available for 'struggling' medical colleagues and the role occupational medicine played. It, however, made me think what fellow medical colleagues had for 'support' around the world; in particular, in Nigeria where I studied and trained as a doctor at Obafemi Awolowo University Teaching Hospitals, Ile-Ife over 25 years ago.

I was really pleased to be awarded the Society of Occupational Medicine Golden Jubilee Travelling Fellowship. My aim was to look at how 'sick doctors' in Nigeria are identified and managed at various stages of their career with a particular emphasis on psychological ill-health. I also took the opportunity to undertake a snapshot prevalence of anxiety and depression using the Hospital Anxiety and Depression Scale (HADS) in training doctors.

I travelled to Nigeria in January 2017 and following a number of introductory meetings with key senior medical academic leads, a number of key themes emerged around poor mental health awareness and the need for early identification and support for medical students and registrars. I subsequently undertook two teaching sessions to scope mental health awareness, the first attended by 18 medical registrars and the second by 64 final year medical students.

The themes that came out of the sessions reflected issues around poor awareness of mental health and associated barriers. The support that was perceived at strategic level did not seem to be reflected among the attendees but it was encouraging to know that there was a perceived need for further work to be done using a more proactive approach. The UK PHP model was well received and it was felt that it was something that could work but the logistics would be a challenge because of the mental health 'stigma' that still exists.

Estimates of the prevalence of mental health problems vary from country to country but in the UK 23% of adults have at least one diagnosed mental health problem at any one point in time. The prevalence in Nigeria has been recorded as being between 45 and 47% in primary care for depression, and as high as 50% for anxiety. Although mine was a very small sample size, the reported prevalence from the attendees was 22% for anxiety and 13% for depression which are both similar to the life time risk from previous research studies. These key findings provided some insights into the lives of the training doctor and were fed back to the medical leadership for both the medical school and the teaching hospital with recommendations. The dean for the medical school has since acknowledged the findings and the recommendations are being fed back to the faculty board and the appropriate actions taken.

Source: *Occupational Medicine*, Volume 67, Issue 6, August 2017, Page 441, https://doi.org/10.1093/occmed/kqx074. Copyright © The Author 2017.

Which way is up?

Mike Gibson

Over 20 years ago, I was an exchange officer in the Office of the US Air Force (USAF) Surgeon General. One task I was given was to evaluate a course run by the Air National Guard (ANG) called 'Top Knife', intended to turn ANG flight surgeons into fighter surgeons. Could it be expanded to USAF flight surgeons and possibly make USAF dentists, who were much more remote from the air aspects of the Air Force, more air minded? To carry out this task, I had to attend the course at Klamath Falls in Oregon. I was the first British officer to participate and only the second 'alien' to do so after an Australian in Air Combat Command.

The course comprised three elements spread over 2 weeks: an academic programme and online examination conducted by the University of Oregon; providing cover for the ANG 114th Tactical Fighter Training Squadron as they were a full-time squadron whose flight surgeon was a weekend warrior; and obtaining flight experience in a fighter plane, the F-16D. Day 1 was administration and familiarization with the academic resources. Day 2 involved kitting out and a trip in the flight simulator, but with the weapons system controls covered because I was an alien. (This was addressed by one of the instructors in the actual aircraft, as I was expected to be able to use the weapons in flight.) Day 3 was foggy so I did the exam, and in the remaining six flying days, I managed 14.5 hours of air combat training.

The pilots I flew with had memorable call signs such as Skull, Gnarly, Ambush, Rocky, Moose, Badger and Maggott; mine was a more prosaic 'Doc'. The safety pilot was not allowed to let me take off or land, but I was cleared to do everything else including air-to-air refuelling, formation aerobatics, intercepts and flying supersonic. The F-16D was cleared to very high levels of gravitational force (g) and the standard drill was to do two high g 'awareness' turns on the way to the range. In air combat, the rate of onset of g was impressive and it needed all our training and equipment to maintain vision during high g. Changes of course and altitude were done routinely by performing a variant of a split-S manoeuvre (half-roll, half-loop up or down, exit in a different direction). I got used to seeing Oregon upside down and I rapidly overcame my initial airsickness. I have never had so much fun in my life.

After I returned to Washington, the Air Attaché in the British Embassy, a professional aviator, was exceedingly jealous and did not speak to me for weeks. Obviously, I recommended the course for the USAF but suggested that the name for the dental participants should be changed from 'Top Knife' to 'Top Gum'. I failed. The course, which still runs, is called 'Top Tooth'.

Source: *Occupational Medicine*, Volume 65, Issue 8, November 2015, Page 650, https://doi.org/10.1093/occmed/kqu093. Copyright © The Author 2015.

Reprinted by permission of Oxford University Press on behalf of the Society of Occupational Medicine.

Tales of Kieran: The occupational physician's odyssey 8—The HAVS and the Have Nots

J.A. Hunter

I was passing the occupational health department the other day and decided to call in. Kieran's door was slightly ajar, so I knocked and pushed it open. The entire floor of his office was covered with large pictures of what looked like people's hands, and there in the middle of all this digital photography was Kieran, crouched on all fours, peering intently at one of the pictures through a magnifying glass.

'You haven't opened up a manicure service now Kieran?' I joked, remembering the aroma-therapy incident.

'Have', came the mumbled response as he leant even closer to the photograph in question.

'You haven't?'

'Haves' I thought he said, louder.

'You have?'

He looked up exasperated. 'HAVES!'

'Haves?' I was starting to wonder if this was some infantile game where I was meant to say 'have not' or something.

'H.A.V.S', he reiterated, as if I was some kind of semi-illiterate. 'Hand Arm Vibration Syndrome.' He turned back to his photographs. 'Can't see any blanching though.'

I mulled HAVS over in my brain. I am sure it had been white finger when I had been at medical school, and whilst times change, HAVS sounds a bit stupid really. Medicine loves its acronyms, but some of the occupational ones are completely incomprehensible, like COSHH or WRULD. And then there is all the management speak they seem to know. I remember the time when Kieran was doing some work for one of the local Japanese implants and all he ever spoke about was karoshi and kaizen and JIT.

'So come on then, Kieran, what has this gallery of hand shots got to do with HAVS, or whatever you call it nowadays?'

Kieran put his glass down and pulled himself up. 'There has been a bit of a glut of HAVS claims from council workers and the council wanted an expert opinion because they were a bit concerned about the legitimacy of some of the diagnoses being made. As a major academic department, they approached me.'

'The diagnosis is quite simple isn't it? Surely, you just stick their hands in cold water, they go white and there's your proof?' I realized I had said the wrong thing as Kieran embarked on a tirade about thermal aesthesiometry, two-point discrimination and how sophisticated the testing was when done under laboratory controlled conditions. I had never realized it was so scientific and was quite impressed.

'So you can make the diagnosis pretty confidently with all these tests then can you?'

'Aaahh, well no, not exactly.' He looked a little uncomfortable at this. 'You see, the sensitivity and specificity of the tests are not very good.'

'You mean that, despite all the sophisticated equipment and testing, the diagnosis rests on the history?'

'Yes, you could say that … as well as the staging of the condition and therefore how much compensation they receive, and more to the point, there are websites giving information about what to say and which peg to drop. It's called patient empowerment I believe.'

'So where does the photography come in?' I could tell I had asked the right thing as a look of pride crept over Kieran's face.

'Well you see, I hit on this idea of giving the claimant a digital camera so that each time they suffered an attack they could take a photograph and we would immediately have a record of when they suffered it, how extensive it was and also the frequency of attacks, because the camera records dates and times automatically, and—this is the clever bit—you would know if they had photographed someone else's hands because they would be different from your reference photograph taken in the clinic.'

'That's brilliant!'

'Yes, I thought so but …'

'But what?'

'So far we have only had two people return the camera out of the fifteen we have offered it to, and I haven't been able to find any blanching at all. I think it might be a case of insufficient pixels?' With a sigh, he got back down on his hands and knees and returned to his task. I decided to leave him to it, but as I left I couldn't help noticing how quite a few photographs were of the index and middle fingers only, and their intended message was pretty obvious from this distance. Whether Kieran will see the subtlety of it with that magnifying glass is another matter.

Source: *Occupational Medicine*, Volume 53, Issue 6, 1 September 2003, Page 416, https://doi.org/10.1093/occmed/kqg124. Copyright © Society of Occupational Medicine 2003.

Reprinted by permission of Oxford University Press on behalf of the Society of Occupational Medicine.

Don Valley festival champions

David Walker

Two things have happened since the adjudicator (Occup Med August 2009;59:362). First, he's not been invited back. Some choristers took his feedback personally. Others felt our musical director had been undermined. Those who enjoyed it and wanted more were in the minority.

Second, we won The Don Valley Festival, a week-long annual music and arts shindig near Barnsley. A large audience, a big cup, a slightly less big cheque and a massive barrel of Eastwood's bitter. It is just the best way of getting feedback: we sounded great, for one performance at least.

Where do we go from here? We don't have a set of targets, which is a relief. We have a hard working committee and a charity mission statement that says something about promoting choral music in the community. A prior informal understanding that we did not do competitions has now gone. As a mixed ability choir, our auditions assess basic skills only. Selection could be one way forward, though not without its problems. My pal Big Dave, twenty stone bass with Cadenza, an Edinburgh Choir, tells me their MD holds strict auditions. She specifically looks for balance, thus excluding, heaven forbid, the rogue distinctive single voice. The confident and consistent outfit we have become is very good for new members, but the new guys do change the balance until they are bedded in.

We are a strong team headed by a first-rate musical director and pianist. Over 60 singers attend a two hour rehearsal once weekly, with extra sectionals once a month. Most turn out for our annual away weekend, currently held in Scarborough. Voice coaching remains a gap. Gordon Shepherd, Ark Occupational Health, tells me that he and some of his barbershop pals go for professional residential singing lessons, expensive but excellent value. Learning occurs in formal sessions and during the afterglow in the bar. Their sections also submit CD recordings to the MD and voice coaches within the choir. Gordon is okay with this, but he admits it is softly, softly at the moment.

In addition to that one performance, what is the evidence for improvement? We are still being invited to appear with other musical ensembles, CD sales are steady, bums on seats at our own concerts are satisfactory to good, small profits are being made and newspaper reviews are favourable. Having great guests is a good tip. Since the adjudicator we have had Aled Jones and Morriston Male Orpheus. Our normal fan base of wives, partners and friends was boosted. The reviews got rosier too.

Can individuals make a difference? Voice coaching is an anatomy lecture, a demonstration and practice, practice, practice. So the answer is yes. But it needs paying for and you get feedback a plenty: good and bad. The evidence for keeping up or getting better? The top choirs have a regular voice test and very few singers look forward to it.

The adjudicator left some bruised egos and a crumb of confidence. We can only get better.

Source: *Occupational Medicine*, Volume 60, Issue 3, May 2010, Page 171, https://doi.org/10.1093/occmed/kqp193. Copyright © The Author 2010.

Why I became an occupational physician …

Ian Reid-Entwistle

Firstly I should explain why I became a doctor. My grandfather was science master at Hindley grammar school in Lancashire about the turn of the last century when with four children he re-entered Manchester University and studied medicine. He funded this course by teaching physics and chemistry at night class, which involved a 12 mile walk. After qualification he worked as an assistant in general practice before serving as medical officer in the trenches in France during World War 1. He had a great interest in shipping and on his half days took me from Bolton to Liverpool where we would travel on the overhead railway and view the merchant shipping in the docks and stately liners alongside the pier head.

My first house job was casualty officer in Liverpool where I established a working relationship with Dr J. Brown then medical superintendent of Cunard. I was enthralled and awestruck when he invited me to dine on board the liner Sylvania. Later, as a junior partner in a general practice, I was able to persuade his successor the irascible Robert Heggie, medical superintendent of the Cunard steamship company, to allow me to act as relief surgeon for a transatlantic voyage to New York in my holiday time. The experience exceeded all my expectations and was repeated annually in the early 1960s, during which time I acted as principal medical officer to various Cunard liners including RMS Mauritania, Queen Mary and Queen Elizabeth. On serving in RMS Carinthia, I transferred a moribund seaman with multiple injuries in an open boat in mid-Atlantic from a Norwegian freighter. I saved the man's life and the case received great publicity. Cunard remembered it when they invited me at the age of 34 to be the fifth medical superintendent in the company's history, a position which I held for 30 years. Initially my remit included that of medical officer to Cunard Eagle International Airways but my most rewarding job with Cunard was to design and equip the hospital in QE2, and subsequently serve and work in my own hospital.

Thus I became an occupational physician and a founder member of the Faculty of Occupational Medicine. As the volume of shipping declined in the 1970s I was able to expand my interest in other industries and I have occupied diverse positions such as performing sessional work for the benefits agency on Merseyside, and establishing and running an occupational medical service for a large national consortium of private hospitals from their flagship hospital in the West End of London. I retired at the age of 76.

During a lifetime of occupational medicine I have been privileged to travel the world and meet and work with an incredible range of human beings, from the very highest and the bravest to the most disadvantaged. It has allowed me, amongst other things, to enjoy a high standard of living and indulge my taste in exotic motorcars, period houses, horticulture and travel.

Source: *Occupational Medicine*, Volume 63, Issue 4, June 2013, Page 305, https://doi.org/10.1093/occmed/kqt016. Copyright © The Author 2013.

Originally from: Entwistle IR. An experience at sea. *Occup Med (Lond)* 1963;**13**:127–131. Accessible online at http://occmed.oxfordjournals.org/content/13/1/127.full.pdf+html

Pegasus at Wanlockhead

Timothy Finnegan

With Pegasus upon a day,
Apollo, weary flying,
Through frosty hills the journey lay,
On foot the way was plying.
Poor slipshod giddy Pegasus
Was but a sorry walker;
To Vulcan then Apollo goes,
To get a frosty caulker.
Obliging Vulcan fell to wark,
Threw by his coat and bonnet,
And did Sol's business in a crack;
Sol paid him with a sonnet.
Ye Vulcan's sons of Wanlockhead,
Pity my sad disaster;
My Pegasus is poorly shod,
I'll pay you like my master.

One of Mike McKiernan's Art and Occupation articles described David Allan's picture of Lead Mining at Leadhills [1]. It brought to my mind Robert Burns's poem Pegasus at Wanlockhead. The Leadhills and Wanlockhead railway is a 2 ft (610 mm) narrow gauge railway in South Lanarkshire, Scotland, laid on the trackbed of the former Leadhills and Wanlockhead Branch of the Caledonian Railway [2]. The original railway closed in the late 1930s shortly after the mines in Wanlockhead had closed. The 'preserved' section runs from Leadhills for about 1 km (0.6 mile) towards Wanlockhead and is the highest adhesion railway in the UK.

The story behind the sonnet reflects Burns's quick wit and erudition. It is a practical, problem-solving poem. Burns was mounted on his new horse, Pegasus, on a frosty afternoon in the winter of 1788–89 and called at the smithy in Wanlockhead. However, the blacksmith was too busy to frost Pegasus's shoes; a frosty caulker or calker is a metal projection on a horseshoe to prevent slipping on ice. It may be enough to just turn over the front edges. Undeterred, Burns and a local acquaintance, Thomas Sloan, went to Ramage's Inn at 3 p.m. There Burns composed the sonnet and addressed it to John Taylor, a man of standing in the community. Taylor spoke to the smith and Pegasus's shoes were frosted. Burns uses mythical allusions to Apollo, the Greek god of poetry and the Sun, and Sol, the ancient Roman Sun god, as himself and Vulcan, the Roman god of metal working, whose symbols were the anvil, tongs and hammer, as the smith. Pegasus, the winged horse of Greek mythology, is more familiar now as the emblem of British airborne forces.

In the 18th century, the blacksmith was one of the most important people in a village. He was the local 'engineer' and had sufficient intellect and business sense to hold a church or legal appointment. His skill as a metal craftsman enabled him to make functional as well as decorative items—tools, horseshoes, wrought iron work—as well as mend metal fixtures and implements. The horse was the motive power not only for farm-work but also for personal mobility and keeping horses mobile was important for the local economy. In 1788, the year before he wrote the poem, Burns travelled on the first steam boat towards the beginning of the Industrial Revolution. Today Wanlockhead is near Junction 14 of the A74(M) and the smithy in the sonnet is now the tourist information office.

References

1. **McKiernan M, David Allan**. Lead Processing at Leadhills, Pounding the Ore c. 1786. *Occup Med (Lond)* 2016;**66**:349–350.
2. Leadhills and Wanlockhead Railway, http://www.leadhillsrailway.co.uk/ (17 February 2017, date last accessed).

Source: *Occupational Medicine*, Volume 67, Issue 7, October 2017, Page 509, https://doi.org/10.1093/occmed/kqx084. Copyright © The Author 2017.

One hundred years of the health and safety laboratory 5

Anon

Nippy was a Buxton site locomotive (Figure 170.1). Wagons of coal would be transported along an embankment by a British railway wagon to a 40 ton bunker close to the coal dust explosion gallery. Here, two to three tonnes of coal would be pulverised in the dust preparation plant, and this would be fed into a dust-laying machine. At this point Nippy came into action, as the SMRE designed dust machine would be hitched to Nippy and be drawn along the gallery, where it would deposit a layer of dust in readiness for a coal dust explosion test. Nippy left the site at some point, but can now be found at the Stradbally Woodland Express Railway, where it is actually the oldest narrow gauge operational diesel loco in Ireland.

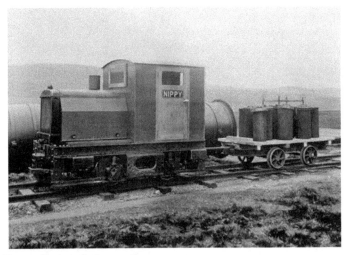

Figure 170.1 Nippy a Buxton site locomotive
© Crown Copyright 2011.

Source: *Occupational Medicine*, Volume 61, Issue 5, August 2011, Page 348, https://doi.org/10.1093/occmed/kqr105. © Crown copyright 2011.

Reprinted by permission of Oxford University Press on behalf of the Society of Occupational Medicine.

Fifty years ago: 'Searching for occupational cancer risks'

Joan M. Davies

There is by now a long list of proven occupational cancer risks; these cover a wide range of jobs and carcinogenic substances, and a variety of cancer sites. One occupational cancer recently brought to light, where the exact agent is not yet known, is carcinoma of the nasal cavity and accessory sinuses in woodworkers. Acheson, Hadfield and Macbeth (1967) examined the incidence of this cancer in men in Oxfordshire and parts of Berkshire and Buckinghamshire and found that from 1956 to 1965, there had been 17 cases among some 12000 woodworkers, although not more than one case would have been expected according to regional age-specific rates. The excess of cases was among furniture workers in High Wycombe. Intensive work is currently being carried out on the cancer mortality of a number of occupational groups including asbestos workers and rubber workers. But there are various suspected occupational cancer risks which still await investigation, and which an industrial medical officer may be well placed to study. For instance, it has long been suspected that metal dust can cause cancer of the larynx, but it seems that nobody has yet taken a group of men with past exposure of this kind and made a survey of their subsequent cancer mortality.

Apart from proven or suspected risks, it is not generally appreciated that there may be many unsuspected cancer risks in our midst that have given rise to unnoticed clusters of occupational cancers of one site or another. Such clusters can all too easily be missed unless someone is on the alert and looking out for them. There is no reliable system of detecting occupational cancer risks—one cannot rely on their being discovered by the Registrar-General's occupational mortality studies, nor by sporadic retrospective surveys of the past occupations of series of cancer patients; cancer registries are not in a position to discover unsuspected occupational hazards, because their information on patients' jobs is very scanty. The people in a position to notice a risk are either factory medical officers or hospital doctors, who may be observant enough to notice that several patients with the same sort of cancer have done the same kind of work—this was how the woodworkers' cancer was first observed. But unless the cancer concerned is a common one like lung or stomach, there may be a large relative excess of cases over what normally occurs in the population—perhaps 10-fold—and yet the actual number of cases will be small—perhaps only one case a year or even less among a factory's past and present employees. One must stress past and present, for occupational cancers are characterized by a long latent period averaging around 20 years between the worker's first exposure to the carcinogen and the subsequent development of the disease. This means that some of the workers affected will have either retired or left to take other jobs before they fall ill; these cases probably never come to the notice of the factory, and at hospital it is the subsequent job that is recorded on their case-notes, or they are just described as 'retired', and the clinician may not notice the connection either. On the other hand, an excess of cases of stomach cancer may not be conspicuous because this is a common cancer anyway, and with cancer of the lung knowledge of the high risk among cigarette smokers may have made people less alert to the occupational aspect (Figure 171.1).

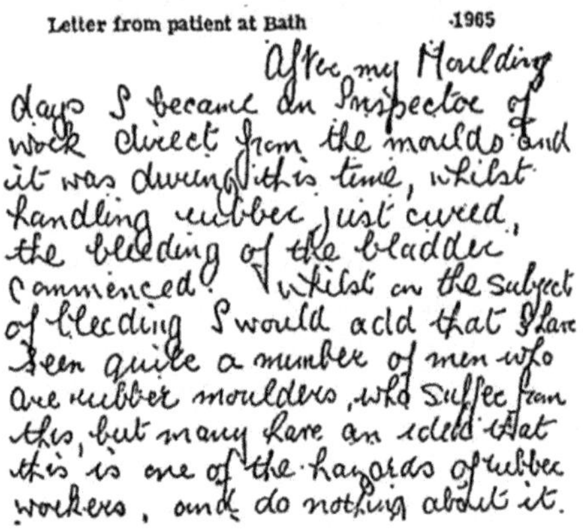

Letter from patient at Bath 1965

Fɪɢ. 1

Part of a letter from a former rubber worker who had been treated for a bladder tumour.

Figure 171.1 Part of a letter from a former rubber worker who had been treated for a bladder tumour.

Reproduced with permission from Searching for occupational cancer risks. (1968). *Trans Soc Occup* Med. 18(1): 42–48. https://doi.org/10.1093/occmed/18.1.42

Source: *Occupational Medicine,* Volume 68, Issue 2, March 2018, Page 155, https://doi.org/10.1093/occmed/kqx193. Copyright © The Author(s) 2018.

Originally from: Searching for occupational cancer risks. *Trans Soc Occup Med* (1968) 18, 42–48. Available at: *Occup Med (Lond)* 1968;18:42–48. DOI:10.1093/occmed/18.1.42

Ready, Fire, Aim!

John Hobson

Early on in my career as an occupational physician, I spent a number of years working for a French multinational company. Once established, I was sent to France for 3 months of company immersion. There were 47 of us, half newly recruited from the grand écoles, the elite of the French educational system. The remainder were experienced managers either from France or foreigners like myself from throughout Europe and America. We were now cadre, the professional elite in an egalitarian republic. All male, we were engineers and production managers, accountants and computer programmers, personnel managers and designers, cartographers and chemists and a doctor.

We had lectures from senior people in the business, we visited factories, we spent time working on the shop floor and experienced research and development and commerce. We were each set a business problem to solve, a project totally unrelated to our professional background and we had to work in small groups to tackle other projects. Everything was conducted in French.

We worked together in an open plan office, groups of four around a desk sharing a telephone. The atmosphere was friendly and cooperative; we ate out at a different restaurant every day and when not working played football and squash, or visited local sites of interest and went skiing. There were company monitors to watch over us, follow our progress and discover the impression we left when we met senior managers. Activity became more frenetic as projects got behind schedule. We were collectively shocked when a couple of the new recruits suddenly disappeared, their desks cleared and their names removed from the notice board.

Gradually cultural differences emerged, seen most starkly in meetings. A 'northern' meeting took place first thing in the morning. It started exactly on time. It also ended at the predetermined time whether the business was finished or not. The proceedings were efficient, all points noted and decisions were made.

A 'southern' meeting often had a staggered start once everybody had turned up. The only thing likely to stop the meeting was lunch or dinner and in between meals le meeting was an open forum for everybody to talk about themselves for as long as possible.

Inevitably the two cultures were unable to adjust to each other. The northern meeting was accused of being a case of Ready, Fire, Aim! They rushed into decisions, usually getting it wrong. The southern meeting preferred to take their time to consider everything, debate it fully and only put it into action when they were sure it would work. The north counter attacked. Even by the time they had held a meeting, made a decision, implemented it, got it wrong and then put it right, the south were still talking about it.

Recent political events have led me to reflect on my European experience. If the diversity did cause difficulties, it was also a strength and my time in France was one of the best experiences of my life and something I will never forget.

Source: *Occupational Medicine*, Volume 67, Issue 1, 1 January 2017, Page 32, https://doi.org/10.1093/occmed/kqw122. Copyright © The Author 2017.

Reprinted by permission of Oxford University Press on behalf of the Society of Occupational Medicine.

Why I became an occupational physician …

Chris Sharp

In 1983, sheltering in a shell-damaged hangar during an artillery battle at Beirut International airport I found myself wondering about my career. I was accompanying a wounded American marine whilst for the first time in my life carrying a loaded pistol with the safety catch off as the RAF Chinook helicopter that had delivered me there, disappeared into the distance. The American helicopter that was meant to be picking us up was late. Having trained in general medicine and latterly in general practice, I joined the RAF partly because of disillusionment with the NHS and partly due to a fascination with aircraft. Whilst the current situation was exciting, and in the emergency medicine connotation appropriate, this was not something I wanted to do for the rest of my career. Three weeks later I found myself landing in the middle of Beirut, again during an artillery battle, with a medic in the middle of the night, to pick up a wounded television sound recordist. Neither of these episodes appeared to be about preventing injury or rehabilitating 'patients'.

My interest in flying had been present from an early age, but my manifest myopia had been a preclusion to starting a flying career in the 1970s. After joining the RAF, I was privileged to be able to fly with the aircrew that I looked after and to be informally trained in flying fixed and rotary wing aircraft. The latter became very real as a skill in Northern Ireland, Cyprus and The Falklands, where I was involved in retrieving casualties, supporting them in flight and delivering them to secondary care. Normally on the return trips to base I would be in control of the aircraft. Subsequently, the RAF formally taught me to fly and I gained my private pilot's licence, partly achieving my ambition.

I completed my first formal occupational medicine course—the Diploma in Aviation Medicine—and acquired skills to assess the capability of aircrew to return to operations after illness and injury. It was one particular aircrew assessment after injury that convinced me that a career in occupational medicine was where my interests would be fulfilled. I had to assess a fighter pilot after musculoskeletal injury. His future flying career would be affected significantly by an adverse assessment and might have condemned him to non-flying duties. Much to his relief, my assessment and report allowed him to return to flying duties, and as it turned out to an interesting future career. This assessment, among others that I completed in my role, confirmed my desire and satisfaction with occupational medicine and led me to apply for formal occupational medicine training. The rest is history as they say and that former pilot is the current world land speed record holder! Partly thanks to him, I have had an amazingly satisfying career, but perhaps in some way I also contributed to the UK holding a world record.

Source: *Occupational Medicine*, Volume 66, Issue 8, November 2016, Page 594, https://doi.org/10.1093/occmed/kqw077. Copyright © The Author 2016.

Reprinted by permission of Oxford University Press on behalf of the Society of Occupational Medicine.

Demoralization and stress—we can all help (?)

Frank Klont

'Finally, it's the weekend!' These words or words to similar effect can be heard quite often in and around our city's university medical centre, and admittedly, these words pass my lips as well occasionally. Most of us will recognize those weeks when nothing comes easy, and we have all probably experienced longing for the weekend when you can clear your mind and recharge your battery. So far nothing unusual or disturbing. Unfortunately, for some of us, longing for the weekend is not a seldomly encountered sensation, but rather a recurring one. Notwithstanding the inspiring, life-changing and even life-saving nature of our jobs, enjoying our work to the fullest may at times feel like an unattainable goal to some. Clearly, we cannot completely control our lives, and we should anticipate encountering difficulties and misfortune in our lives. Occasional setbacks may even be considered beneficial as they may help you to realize how good life can be. Nonetheless, one may wish to apply the dictum of Paracelsus 'dosis sola facit venenum' (freely translated as the dose determines whether something is harmful) to facing difficulties, and regularly experiencing longing for the weekend may be a symptom of an impaired state of mind.

As a reader of Occupational Medicine, you are likely to be confronted with work-related stress and mental health problems on a regular basis, and you may have helped many individuals to regain a positive attitude. However, these mental health issues are probably not just present in those who seek help; some people in need of support may leave it too late to knock on your door, or do not even dare to do so at all. Therefore, I would like to suggest that we all, professionals and non-professionals, keep an ear to the ground to recognize signs of discomfort in good time. And when we encounter such signs, let us (try to) talk with and listen to those in discomfort, and encourage them to talk and listen as well. Allow them to convince themselves of the (unfortunate) commonness of their feelings of demoralization as well as of the importance of opening up about these feelings, to themselves, to people around them, and possibly also to health care professionals. Together we can contribute to tackling mental health stigma by encouraging openness about mental health problems and by stimulating positive attitudes towards help-seeking. Together, we may contribute to relieving the overall burden of dissatisfaction with work and burnout by helping unhappy individuals to seek the support they need in time. Because in the end, let us not forget how great life is, how great life can be and how it is important to celebrate it all, even when 'Finally, it's Monday!'

Source: *Occupational Medicine*, Volume 68, Issue 1, January 2018, Page 17, https://doi.org/10.1093/occmed/kqx140. Copyright © The Author(s) 2018.

Reprinted by permission of Oxford University Press on behalf of the Society of Occupational Medicine.

Keeping hat making alive in Luton

Kirstie Gibson

Before the Second World War, most people wore hats most of the time. The hat symbolized social status and work trade, examples being the bowler hat of the civil servant and city worker and the straw boater of the fishmonger and butcher [1]. The decline of hat wearing in the 1960s appears to be linked to the development of the motor vehicle where people did not need head protection from the elements and wearing a hat in modern vehicles is inconvenient [2]. There have been recent resurgences of hat wearing in the general male population with baseball caps and a new generation of flat cap wearers in younger men, although women's hat wearing is still largely restricted to sun hats and religious and social events like weddings [3].

The Luton and Dunstable area has been the centre of hat making for over 200 years and started with straw hats that were probably developed in Italy and came to England in the 1600s [4]. The straw hat is made from a long length of straw plait that is sewn together to make a hat. The hat is shaped on a block, dyed, strengthened with shellac or gelatine and finished with lining and a ribbon trimming. Straw plaiting was undertaken by hand mostly by women and young girls working at home. They would plait all day and make an 18 metre long plait. There were high levels of child labour and children were sent to a plait school aged 3 or 4 years old; the schools were more like workshops with little general education available. Older children were expected to produce 27 metres a day. Conditions were cold and cramped and children developed sore lips from licking the straw. The 1867 Workshop Regulation Act banned the employment of children less than 8 years of age and required children from the ages of 8 to 13 to attend school for 10 hours a week. It was difficult for factory inspectors to enforce the law in the Luton area until 1875 [4].

The development of a sewing machine to sew the plait improved productivity and there were many small workshops set up in houses as the start-up costs for equipment were low and profits from a cheap raw product were high. The architecture of Luton demonstrates this with many houses having workshops behind the main house and side gates for horse drawn carts to bring in the raw material [4]. Wool felt hat making developed later in Luton in 1870 to provide more stability in what had been a seasonal industry. After the First World War, the production of felt hats expanded and replaced straw hats and in 1939 made up more than 75% of the Luton hat trade. In the 1930s, it is estimated the area produced 70 million hats a year.

References

1. **Harrison M.** *The History of the Hat.* 1st edn. London: Herbert Jenkins Ltd, 1969; 172.
2. http://www.fashion-era.com/hats-hair/hats_hair_1_wearing_hats_fashion_history.htm.
3. http://news.bbc.co.uk/1/hi/8074663.stm.
4. **Carmichael K, McOmish D, Grech D.** *The Hat Industry of Luton and its Buildings.* 1st edn. Swindon: English Heritage, 2013; 1, 25, 51.

Source: *Occupational Medicine*, Volume 66, Issue 1, January 2016, Page 78, https://doi.org/10.1093/occmed/kqv181. Copyright © The Author 2015.

Reprinted by permission of Oxford University Press on behalf of the Society of Occupational Medicine.

The silent killer

Anthony Seaton

Each one of them has left a wound on my heart. The first was the most awful. I was a final year student doing a locum in paediatrics, on evening casualty duty. The ambulance brought in two pink, sleeping babies and a distraught baby sitter. Nothing could be done; they were dead, a leaking gas fire. It was my first experience of carbon monoxide poisoning. At that time the usual cause was attempted suicide by gas oven or car exhaust in the garage, and anyone on casualty duty became familiar with the condition. Conversion to North Sea gas and the fitting of catalytic converters to vehicles have reduced the risk from these methods. Nevertheless, episodes still occur and many are industrial accidents. All are preventable.

The most recent was a lady who had a demanding job requiring numeracy and communication skills. She also had a hobby, at which she was a national expert, requiring frequent travel. In order to reduce her energy bills she arranged to have her roof insulated. Unfortunately a pump the workers brought was sited next to a vent into her house. When her carbon monoxide alarm went off she was assured that it was just a fault and switched it off but just before she lost consciousness, she managed to make a confused call to her mother who was able to get an ambulance. Thanks to sympathetic management by her employer she eventually got back to work but her brain damage means she can never perform this at other than a very basic level. Her hobby is lost to her. Her life is destroyed.

When I say that these accidents are preventable I imply that in Britain we have systems that reduce risk. In less advanced countries I have often seen good regulation but poor or absent enforcement, and I used to be confident that here we were better at making sure the regulations were adhered to. Two things seem to have happened that make me feel less confident. First, industries have changed and now we have either very large companies where those at the top have little idea of what goes on at the bottom, or very small concerns where the owners are ignorant of health and safety issues and confident that they are unlikely to be bothered by an overstretched inspectorate. Secondly, we have seen a systematic denigration of 'Health 'n' Safety', part of an attempt to free industry of red tape and make us prosperous again.

I know I am biased since I only see patients when something has gone wrong, but I do feel that a nation has lost its soul when it ceases to care about the workers who, after all, support our economy. Tennyson described nature as 'red in tooth and claw'. This describes unregulated capitalism also; Adam Smith's invisible hand is no use against predators. Only red tape, strong and tightly bound, can control them. But where do we hear the call for more of it?

Source: *Occupational Medicine*, Volume 63, Issue 6, September 2013, Page 392, https://doi.org/10.1093/occmed/kqt088. Copyright © The Author 2013.

Why I might become an occupational physician

Joshua Devonport

As part of my fourth year at medical school, I completed a 4-week placement with an occupational health (OH) service provider. The purpose of the placement was to explore occupational medicine as a career by observing occupational physicians and other OH professionals and gain an insight into the specialty. I chose the placement because it offered a specialty to which there was no exposure during my medical training.

The first thing that impressed me was the range of opportunities within occupational medicine. Whilst working with one OH provider, I was exposed to a broad range of industries and work places. Such variety brought to light the breadth of knowledge required from the OH physician. A particular point of interest involved a tour of a truck tyre retreading factory which demonstrated how important it is that occupational physicians possess a good understanding of the work environment and role of the employees with whom they consult.

A significant point of contrast was the duration of consultations; new referrals could take up to an hour when including the report writing. This was something that particularly appealed to me as there were no instances where the consultation felt rushed; everybody had a chance to express themselves fully and this removed a frustration I've witnessed in some NHS outpatient clinics. An aspect of the consultations I suspect may be challenging is the altered dynamic of the doctor–patient relationship due to the introduction of a third party: the client on behalf of whom the employee is being seen. It wasn't clear to me how acting in the patient's best interest was necessarily the same as acting in the employer's best interest although I now understand the importance of work in determining health and well-being. In the same regard, report writing often seemed challenging, as their contents were accessible by all parties involved and needed to be written accordingly.

Another part of the specialty I might find challenging is the move toward a primarily advisory role. Whilst diagnosis is still utilized, it is not to the extent of hospital specialities or general practice. Time spent in OH once I've worked as a hospital doctor would afford me a clearer understanding of the degree to which such an adjustment might impact. One of the most appealing attributes of occupational medicine for me was the regular hours and resulting work–life balance: a feeling that was echoed by all the OH practitioners I met. This could be important when it comes to applying for jobs.

Although it is some years before I can apply for an ST3 post in occupational medicine, this placement provided an enjoyable introduction to the specialty that I would otherwise not have experienced. Occupational medicine is certainly something I will consider as a career. All the physicians I met were enthusiastic about the specialty and happy to answer my questions and a placement such as this is something I would thoroughly recommend to any medical student interested in finding out more about occupational medicine.

Source: *Occupational Medicine*, Volume 66, Issue 9, 19 December 2016, Page 697, https://doi.org/10.1093/occmed/kqw139. Copyright © The Author 2016.

Occupational eye hazard of renaissance sculptor Benvenuto Cellini and the recurrent theme of Pigeon's blood

Timo Hannu

Benvenuto Cellini (1500–71), an Italian sculptor, is known for his bronze sculpture 'Perseus with the Head of Medusa', which is now located in the Loggia dei Lanzi in Florence. Cellini also wrote a famous autobiography in which the following occupational eye injury is described [1] occurring when Cellini worked with his sculpture 'Narcissus' in the 1540s.

"One morning I was preparing some small chisels for my work on it, and an extremely fine splinter of steel flew into my right eye, and it was so far embedded into my pupil that I could not find a way to remove it. I thought for certain that I would lose the sight of that eye. After several days I summoned Master Raffaello de' Pilli, a surgeon who took two live pigeons, and making me lie on my back on a table, he took the pigeons, and with a little knife, pierced a large vein they have in their wings so that the blood ran into my eye; I immediately felt relief as a result, and in the space of two days the steel splinter came out and I remained free of pain and my vision improved."

The type of Cellini's ocular injury was most likely a superficial corneal foreign body. It is unclear how common this type of injury was in the Renaissance, but nowadays it is the most common occupational ocular trauma associated particularly with grinding [2], a work Cellini was performing before the injury. No contemporary practitioner of medicine would suggest using living pigeon's blood but it has been used as a treatment since antiquity and is found as a remedy for eye diseases in Naturalis Historia by Pliny the Elder (d. 79) [3]. Fresh pigeon's blood, especially as a cure for eye injuries, is also mentioned in De Materia Medica by Dioscorides (d. 90) [4], which was the principal book on herbs and other remedies in Europe for over 1500 years.

The unifying theoretical principle for these remedies was provided by Galen (b. 129) in his doctrines of humoral medicine [5]. Treatment consisted of finding a medicine with qualities that counterbalanced the disease. Since the eye itself was considered a phlegmatic organ (cold and wet), the blood of the pigeon would balance the humors. Interestingly, Cellini does not mention the use of forceps, although Byzantine physician Aetios Amidinos (d. 574) wrote in one of his books that forceps should be used to extract small foreign bodies from the eye [6]. Afterwards, dove's blood should be poured onto the injured eye. Instructions for using pigeon's blood can even be found in late 17th century recipe books, which included not only culinary but also medical information. In Lady Ayscough's recipe book from 1692, pigeon's blood is suggested "For A stroke in the Eyes if there Grow pain thereby or if you be pricked in ye Eyes by any thing" [7].

References

1. **Cellini B.** *My Life. Translated by Julia Conaway Bondanella and Peter Bondanella*. New York: Oxford University Press, 2009; 323.
2. **Thompson GJ, Mollan SP.** Occupational eye injuries: a continuing problem. *Occup Med (Lond)* 2009;59:123–125.

3. Pliny the Elder. Cures for eye diseases. In: Natural History, Volume VIII: Books 28–32. Translated by W. H. S. Jones. Loeb Classical Library 418. Cambridge, MA: Harvard University Press, 1963; 263–264.

4. Pedanius Dioscorides of Anazarbus. De materia medica. Translated by Lily Y. Beck. Hildesheim: Olms-Weidmann, 2005; 123.

5. **Siraisi NG.** *Medieval and Early Renaissance Medicine.* Chicago: University of Chicago Press, 1990; 145.

6. **Fronimopoulos J, Lascaratos J.** "Eye injuries" by the Byzantine writer Aetios Amidinos. *Doc Ophthalmol* 1988;**68**:121–124.

7. Lady Ayscough's recipe book of 1692. Manuscript 1026/30, Wellcome Library. London, UK.

Source: *Occupational Medicine*, Volume 68, Issue 2, March 2018, Page 142, https://doi.org/10.1093/occmed/kqx176. Copyright © The Author(s) 2018.

Reprinted by permission of Oxford University Press on behalf of the Society of Occupational Medicine.

Fifty years ago: 'Pulmonary function tests in asbestos workers'

G.L. Leathart

In established asbestosis, examination reveals crepitations at the lung bases, clubbing of the fingers and cyanosis. The clubbing and cyanosis are late and inconstant features, but basal crepitations are nearly always present. To begin with they are fine and are heard at the end of inspiration when the lungs are fully expanded, but as the disease progresses, they become coarser and are audible at lower lung volumes, eventually being heard throughout inspiration. Characteristically they appear first in the axillary basal region but eventually spread throughout the lung. They are heard first at the lung bases because of the effect of gravity. When a patient is examined lying on one side, the crepitations often disappear from the upper lung and are heard only in the lower lung, and this phenomenon is repeated when the patient turns on to the other side. They are heard at the back when the patient is supine and at the front when he is prone. A probable reason for the variations in timing of the crepitations is that the diseased part of the lung is less compliant than the rest and is the last to expand on inspiration, hence delaying the crepitations until the end of inspiration. The postural effects are clinical expressions of the principle that the lowermost part of the lung collapses furthest on expiration and expands most on inspiration (Milic-Emili, Henderson, Dolovich, Trop and Kaneko, 1966). Early in the disease, the crepitations are intermittent, but can sometimes be brought to light by examining the lower lung in a patient lying on one side, or by examining the back of the patient who is supine. The angle between the seat and the head-rest of a hospital examination couch affords a gap through which the back of a supine patient can be reached. Although crepitations are usually present in asbestosis, they are not invariable and a few patients have been seen in whom they were absent despite a positive diagnosis by lung biopsy. In Figure 179.1, the time at which basal crepitations were first heard is indicated by a thickening of the lines, continuous when they were invariably present, interrupted when they were intermittent. This sign was present in five of the subjects and in all of them it was first noted before the diffusing capacity had dropped significantly. Crepitations were not present, however, in two of the cases with a low diffusing capacity, an experience similar to that of Williams and Hugh-Jones (1960). Other measurements made in these 12 subjects showed small and inconsistent changes over the years. Compliance rose on average by 26%, while vital capacity fell by 7–8% during the period of observation.

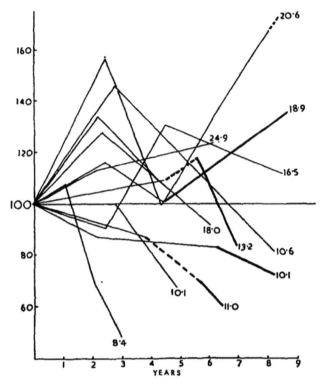

Figure 179.1 Diffusing capacity against time in 12 laggers without asbestosis, expressed as a percentage of the initial observation. Each line represents the progress of a single subject. The figures at the ends of the lines are the final readings in ml./min./mm.Hg

Reproduced with permission from Leathart G. L. (1968). Pulmonary function tests in asbestos workers. *Trans Soc Occup Med.* **18**: 49–55. DOI:10.1093/occmed/18.1.49

Source: *Occupational Medicine*, Volume 68, Issue 3, April 2018, Page 198, https://doi.org/10.1093/occmed/kqx194. Copyright © The Author(s) 2018.

Originally from: Pulmonary function tests in asbestos workers. *Trans Soc Occup Med* (1968) 18, 49–55. Available at: *Occup Med (Lond)* 968;18:49–55.

Reprinted by permission of Oxford University Press on behalf of the Society of Occupational Medicine.

It's not all hot air

Mike Gibson

I have now been playing the bagpipes for almost 60 years. I first became interested in the medical aspects of piping at medical school and later had the opportunity to research the physiological aspects at the RAF Institute of Aviation Medicine.

There is an old joke that pipers march up and down because it is harder to hit a moving target. Whilst that may, or may not, be true, there is a physiological benefit to marching in this way. The combination of hyperventilation and increased intrathoracic pressure can lead to fainting, particularly in young and inexperienced pipers. Keeping on the move facilitates return of blood to the heart by exercising the muscle pump. However, there are other occupational hazards to playing the Highland bagpipes.

Pipers can develop noise-induced hearing loss—although my wife complains that I have a listening deficit, not a hearing deficit. Many years ago, I took my pipes into an anechoic chamber to measure just how noisy they were. The noise at the left ear was 112 dBA (others have measured even higher levels) which is presumably why the HSE recommends hearing protection for pipers in pipe bands. There is a school of thought that those pipers in a band who are near to the drummers, who can be even louder, are more at risk than those in the front rank.

There has been a case of a young piper suffering a pneumothorax when playing, caused by the bursting of a bulla. Other pipers, particularly those who have been immunologically compromised, have been infected by the hide bag. Such bags are traditionally seasoned or kept supple and airtight by syrup or sugar solutions or commercially available seasonings. These are ideal culture media for such 'bag bugs' as cryptococcus or aspergillus, particularly if the piper is a 'wet blower'. Many pipers have moved to Goretex bags which removes the requirement for seasoning and reduces the risk.

One further risk is one not experienced by the author but known to Shakespeare. Shylock says in Act IV of *The Merchant of Venice*, 'And men there are ... when the bagpipe sings i' th' nose cannot contain their urine'.

Source: *Occupational Medicine*, Volume 66, Issue 4, June 2016, Page 291, https://doi.org/10.1093/occmed/kqv209. Copyright © The Author 2016.

Why I became an occupational physician …

Douglas Scarisbrick

I didn't actually set out to become an 'occupational physician'. In 1970, I answered an advertisement for a doctor with the National Coal Board (NCB) in South Wales; but I had no concept of a specialist dealing with the 'world of work' in general. I was a general practitioner in an urban area; we had full lists and there was no deputizing service. Busy nights and weekends on call were followed by full surgeries and lists of home visits the next day. There was little time or energy left for social activities and I knew my job impinged adversely on my family. I was also dissatisfied and uneasy because I was aware that there were holes in my medical knowledge; I felt that as a family doctor, I should have a working knowledge of the whole of medicine, something I felt unable to achieve.

In what was perhaps a subconscious response to this unease, I had taken up a half-day clinical assistantship in the local chest clinic. There my feeling that the demands of general practice were too wide for me was confirmed. But I enjoyed learning more about respiratory conditions, including the ability to make sense of a chest x-ray.

Returning to hospital medicine and gaining a specialist qualification was not an option, but the NCB job advert suggested a possible way out; I had never been near a coal mine, but I knew that miners suffered chest diseases and I had heard of pneumoconiosis. Perhaps the little knowledge of respiratory diseases I had picked up in the chest clinic would provide an entree to an area of work where such conditions were prevalent.

And so it turned out. As a deputy area medical officer in the NCB's medical service, I was one of 40 or so full-time doctors. We were members of a relatively small band of 'industrial medical officers', mainly in the heavy and dirty industries.

I dealt with all the conditions miners were subject to, minor injuries and the after effects of more serious ones, skin conditions and of course chest problems. Miners with radiographic evidence of pneumoconiosis were referred by the medical officers in charge of radiological services (MOsRS), who read the chest x-rays of mine workers under the NCB's periodic x-ray scheme (PXR). After a couple of years, a vacancy for an MORS arose covering the north east of England and Scotland and I was glad to accept the invitation to train for and undertake this role.

I subsequently broadened my experience of industrial medicine, but returned to take responsibility for the medical surveillance of those exposed to harmful dusts at work. Deep coal mining has recently come to an end in the UK, and that is no doubt a good thing, for all those involved and for society at large. But I am glad I had the opportunity to be an industrial medical officer in one of the significant industries of modern times.

Source: *Occupational Medicine*, Volume 67, Issue 3, 1 April 2017, Page 187, https://doi.org/10.1093/occmed/kqx013. Copyright © The Author 2017.

Visit the workplace? What's wrong with it?

Arun Chind

It was the human resources (HR) lady on the phone. I was at the clinic room in a factory, 'doing a list' for hand-arm vibration syndrome. I got the uneasy feeling that by making the request, I was seeking to break a local tradition of clinician insulation from the workplace. 'I am required to visit the workplace and see the workers at work', I explained, '… it's part of health surveillance'. A short write up and a binary ruling of 'fit' or 'unfit' was really what management was after. There were not meant to be any twists to the oft told tale … and surely no role for an Oliver asking for more. What the Dickens was I trying to do?

Only a few minutes previously, I was taking the worker's work history and making little progress with my understanding of what he actually did that exposed his hands to vibration effects. 'I don't know why I am here', summarized the man. That almost made two of us. 'I do pressure testing', he continued … 'that doesn't have any vibration! And I wear gloves'. Parroting Ramazzini's 'and what job do you do' just wouldn't suffice. Boots on the ground (and other PPE), it would have to be.

The marketing department of the occupational health provider with whom I was contracting had set up the clinic. Needless to add, I could not get my mitts on a risk assessment of the worker's duties. I was supposed 'to (just) do the clinic' and send in a report. Causation of consternation (to workers, managers or HR) was off the script.

Workers do like to be left alone. The workload of the day would still await the worker after his clinical consultation with me. There was no one available to take me around, said the HR lady ringing back. Sensing my unease, my worker offered to take me round himself and the HR lady allowed this.

The unofficial tour proved worthwhile. Back in his workplace, the worker was more forthcoming. On some days, he was assigned to polishing pipe fittings using a pneumatic rotary grinder. His regular duties of pressure testing involved dipping metal parts in a water bath looking for bubbles of leaking air as the pressure was raised to the designated psi. The gloves he was wearing as he demonstrated his tasks were thin nitrile. 'The water becomes very cold especially in winter. I've told them to do something about it', he sighed. His symptoms now made sense. I gave him advice and made my recommendations to management.

In the course of our duties, as we walk the walk, we must also talk the talk (and document this). Our involvement must go beyond marvelling at the wonders of the workplace ('And what big eyes you have grandma!') on a guided tour. It pays to be ever watchful and wary of the wolf of workplace peril. As occupational physicians, we do have a lot riding on what's in the 'hood (and also, under it)!

Source: *Occupational Medicine*, Volume 68, Issue 2, March 2018, Page 153, https://doi.org/10.1093/occmed/kqx105. Copyright © The Author(s) 2018.

Why doctors need to be careful with social media

Nerys Williams

The term social media describes web-based applications that enable users to create and share content or to participate in social networking [1]. The term includes 'blogs' such as Twitter, internet forums such as those on www.doctors.net, content communities such as YouTube and social networking sites such as Facebook and LinkedIn.

The terms are familiar but the blurring between public and private presence has meant some doctors' social media comments have come to the notice and sanction from their professional regulator.

GMC guidance on the use of social media is clear [2]. The standard expected of doctors is no different when communicating using these new methods than via face to face or through traditional media.

It advises doctors that social media sites cannot guarantee confidentiality whatever privacy settings are in place, and that whatever you post is visible to your patients, colleagues, employer and the regulator. It warns that photographs may contain embedded information on location which others could view, and that once material is published online it is difficult to remove, can be forwarded by viewers or commented on in a disparaging way.

Both the British Medical Association (BMA) [3] and the Royal College of General Practitioners (RCGP) [4] have also produced guidance for doctors on their social media use, the latter also publishing a 'social media highway code' which contains more detailed advice. A key piece of advice from the BMA is to be aware, follow any employer's policy on social media and to also follow GMC guidance if taking photographs of patients or in workplaces.

The risks associated with inappropriate use of social media are not theoretical. A *British Medical Journal (BMJ)* freedom of information request to the GMC [5] identified that between 1 January 2015 and 30 June 2017 the regulator closed 28 investigations on doctors' use of social media. Fourteen cases were closed without further action being taken, and a further four were closed with advice being issued to the doctor.

Of those which progressed further, three doctors received a warning from the GMC, three doctors were referred to their employers and two doctors had their registration suspended as the result of an investigation. In a further case, the doctor was issued with an undertaking (an agreement between the GMC and the doctor about their future practice), and in another, the doctor was issued with a condition on their registration. Not all modes of social media were represented equally: 20 investigations were into the use of Facebook, six related to use of Twitter, three related to use of WhatsApp, and in one case both Twitter and Facebook use was the source of enquiry.

Complaints had been made by someone acting in a public capacity (someone working for an employer or public body) in over 50% of cases; seven cases were initiated by a member of the public, and six were made by individuals/organizations labelled as 'other', or were the doctors' own self-reports.

Occupational physicians need to be aware of the guidance from the regulator and professional bodies on the use of social media and resist the temptation to feel secure in what is a public forum.

A wise axiom might be that if you wouldn't do it or say it in the workplace to colleagues, staff and clients, then don't say it on social media!

References

1. Oxford University Press. LEXICO. 'Social media'. https://en.oxforddictionaries.com/definition/social_media (3 March 2018, date last accessed).
2. General Medical Council. Doctors' Use of Social Media. London. https://www.gmc-uk.org/guidance/ethical_guidance/21186.asp (3 March 2018, date last accessed).
3. British Medical Association. Social Media, Ethics and Professionalism. London, 2013. https://www.bma.org.uk/advice/employment/ethics/social-media-guidance-for-doctors (3 March 2018, date last accessed).
4. Royal College of General Practitioners London. Social Media Highway Code. 2013. http://www.rcgp.org.uk/social-media (3 March 2018, date last accessed).
5. **Rimmer A.** Doctors' use of Facebook, Twitter, and WhatsApp is the focus of 28 GMC investigations. *Br Med J* 2017;**358**:j4099.

Source: *Occupational Medicine*, Volume 68, Issue 5, July 2018, Page 331, https://doi.org/10.1093/occmed/kqy064. Copyright © The Author(s) 2018.

Reprinted by permission of Oxford University Press on behalf of the Society of Occupational Medicine.

One hundred years of the health and safety laboratory 6

Anon

The picture (Figure 184.1) shows a demonstration of a "triggered water barrier" for suppressing explosions in coal mines. Such explosions, whether through burning methane ('firedamp') or coal dust, can run along a mine roadway burning new gas or dust - possibly for many hundreds of metres. They are a severe risk to miners, and the further the explosion propagates the worse the consequences. The original 'Home Office Experimental Station' was set up to study this kind of explosion and how to reduce its severity. By the time of the photograph, SMRE was still working on developing the state of the art for suppressing such explosions. The triggered barrier was a water filled tube designed to sit in the mine roadway. It had a detector system to spot an explosion coming towards it, which triggered a small charge that forced the water out under pressure. When the explosion reached the location of the barrier, the roadway was filled by a curtain of water that effectively put it out. One concern was that if the barrier was triggered, anyone nearby might be injured by the force of the water. This was of particular concern because you wanted to err on the side of false triggers rather than missing an explosion, so that they might go off in response to something less catastrophic than an explosion. SMRE were sure that the barrier wouldn't cause injuries and the demonstration in the picture was carried out to show how safe it was.

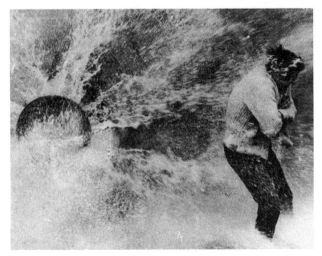

Figure 184.1 Triggered water barrier
© Crown Copyright 2011.

Source: *Occupational Medicine*, Volume 61, Issue 5, August 2011, Page 373, https://doi.org/10.1093/occmed/kqr112. © Crown copyright 2011.

I never knew

John Hobson

I'd worked with her for over 20 years and yet I never knew. When she announced her retirement it felt like the end of an era. During one of our last dinners as working colleagues she told me she had recently been to Stockholm during Nobel Prize presentation week. As a child she remembered going to the Nobel Prize dinner and sitting on a table with other small children, one of whom was now the King of Sweden. To relive memories of attending the awards ceremony all those years before she had gone to the Nobel Museum, which displays the details of all the Nobel Prize winners since 1901. 'That's my father,' she said, showing me a photograph of a display in the museum 'and that's my grandfather,' showing me another. I had to ask her to repeat this a few times. She had never mentioned this in all the years I had known her. 'I wanted people to accept me for who I was rather than someone from a family with two Nobel Prize winners. The only time it became known was when my father died. I had been visiting him repeatedly in Cambridge and when his obituary was published someone put two and two together because of my surname. Fortunately I persuaded them to keep the information to themselves.'

Her grandfather, Sir Henry Dale, together with Otto Loewi, won the 1936 Nobel Prize for medicine for the discovery of acetylcholine. As a medical student, Dale was infamously involved and implicated in the Brown Dog Affair having allegedly killed the dog after the experiments had been concluded. The resulting uproar led to the Brown Dog riots where a thousand medical students carrying effigies of brown dogs on sticks clashed with suffragettes, trades unionists and 400 police officers. Whilst this work led to the discovery of hormones, it also proved a landmark event in the anti-vivisection movement. Dale later became President of the Royal Society.

Her father won the 1957 Nobel Prize for Chemistry for his research on the structure and synthesis of nucleotides, nucleosides and coenzymes. His career was arguably even more illustrious than that of his father-in-law; he received 40 honorary degrees, was created a life peer and was also president of the Royal Society. He also chaired the Royal Commission on Medical Education in the 1960s which recommended that occupational medicine and public health should be made specialities.

Like her father and grandfather, she had strong links to Cambridge but despite a strong sense of loyalty she enjoyed our meetings in Oxford very much. During all that time I never knew that the person who was so influential in our speciality for 20 years had a family which included not one but two Nobel Prize winning Presidents of the Royal Society, something possibly unique in British history. Did my admiration for Lord Todd's daughter, Hilary, change when I found out? No, she had always been a remarkable person, she just happened to have a very remarkable family.

Source: *Occupational Medicine*, Volume 67, Issue 9, December 2017, Page 695, https://doi.org/10.1093/occmed/kqx142. Copyright © The Author(s) 2017.

Reprinted by permission of Oxford University Press on behalf of the Society of Occupational Medicine.

Why I became an occupational physician ...

Arun Peter Chind

Growing up in India, the oil-fired furnace next door supplied my lungs with smoke and my dad's engineer colleagues home-tutored and inspired me. Whilst at school I visited fireclay factories, fertilizer works, heavy engineering companies, railway yards, ship and navy yards. I travelled not just on the footplate (strongly recommended for rail physicians) but also on the buffers of overcrowded trains (definitely not recommended). Industrial (and non-industrial) injuries and illnesses were never far away. After medical school I trained in general surgery, passed the FRCS and after moving to the UK, worked in urology, accident and emergency, psychiatry, intensive care medicine, haematology and oncology. Throughout all this, I maintained an unreasonable interest in mathematics and statistics, chemistry, physics, engineering, computing and social sciences. With personal interest, skill profile and work experience like this, there was only one specialty that held a future for me.

I started work in occupational health in October 2012 and due to previous experience as a reviewer, I quickly became a reviewer for this journal. After less than a year at Addenbrooke's Hospital, I completed the diploma and moved to work in industry. I continued to pursue training and certification both in occupational health and occupational hygiene in the UK and abroad (USA, Ireland and Canada), combining full time work with back-to-back training courses. Shortly after achieving MFOM in 2015, I decided to set up my own company to give myself the freedom and reward of self-employment. In 2016 I completed the Industrial Hygiene Technician qualification from the University of North Carolina and became a guest researcher in occupational health and industrial hygiene at the Respiratory Health Division, NIOSH, Morgantown. Later that year, I completed the accelerated (of course!) Master of Public Health from the University of Florida. In 2017, I passed modules in UK employment law & practice. I have coined the phrase 'Extreme CPD' to describe this lifestyle.

My years in occupational health have been a whirlwind of change, challenge, hard graft and progress. Last year, my practice went international, with US-based organizations commissioning independent medical examinations for their UK-based employees. To me, the best part of being an occupational and environmental physician is the core duty to be objective and impartial. More widely, I appreciate the unique role that we can play in being agents of social change and health improvement. We may not earn as much as surgeons, our reports may not always be acceptable to the employee, employer (or both) and our work sometimes goes unappreciated. It nevertheless remains interesting to receive letters written in coherent prose, contesting an opinion on fitness due to "inability to concentrate" but a letter of genuine appreciation from an employee or human resources goes towards redressing this. In my experience, all parties sooner or later, learn to respect and value integrity. Our ability as a speciality, to contend with a diverse range of health conditions, over varied work environments and provide clarity to allow stakeholders find a way forward, makes it all worthwhile.

Source: *Occupational Medicine*, Volume 67, Issue 6, August 2017, Page 412, https://doi.org/10.1093/occmed/kqx080. Copyright © The Author 2017.

Reprinted by permission of Oxford University Press on behalf of the Society of Occupational Medicine.

The early working life of one occupational physician in the 1970s

Eric Teasdale

I joined ICI's Medical Service, as it was then called, in 1976 after completing a three-year general practice vocational training course. ICI offered comprehensive training and it was indeed provided. At the time ICI had many divisions and owned many companies around the world. To name just a few, the divisions were Mond, Organics (formerly Dyestuffs), Agriculture, Petrochemicals, Paints, Plastics, Plant Protection, Fibres and Pharmaceuticals. The site I worked on in Scotland had parts of Organics and Petrochemicals Divisions, plus the major part of Nobel's Explosive Company. On-site manufacture included initiating explosives (detonators), burning explosives (black powder or gunpowder—the stuff which used to be in penny bangers) and blasting explosives (dynamite, sometimes known as gelignite). There was no manufacture of TNT on site.

There were 33 full-time doctors, of the medical variety, in ICI in the UK at the time; Nobel's had many staff with PhDs but they were known as 'Dynamite Doctors'! The Medical Service was charged with looking after staff of which there were 60 000 in the UK alone. ICI employed many more doctors around the world, many nurses, physiotherapists, radiographers, dentists and opticians-to prescribe and dispense safety glasses.

What I hadn't realized at the time is that the job of an occupational physician is defined by the type of organization in which they work and also, very much, by the local culture. Some organizations merely want to abide by legislative requirements, whereas others realize the importance of having a happy, healthy workforce to maximize innovation, creativity and, ultimately, productivity. Within ICI the Medical Service provided a clinical service, information on the toxicity of the materials handled, and an industrial hygiene service with a focus on dust, noise and fume. It also carried out epidemiology studying the effects of work and working practices on human health.

My time in Scotland provided a valuable introduction to occupational medicine. Accidents were fortunately rare but, when they occurred often resulted in major injury and, on one occasion, death. Accidents were almost always the result of human error and failure to operate 'Safe Systems of Work'. When, after just short of 5 years, I transferred to ICI's Pharmaceuticals Division, the problems were of an entirely different nature. Staff were often employed for their scientific knowledge and skills to discover and develop medicines for human use. It was as if they were employed for what they had from the neck upwards—their brains. It took some years for the industry to realize that physical health, from the neck downwards, was also important to ensure that members of staff could maintain a high level of innovation, creativity and productivity week after week, month after month and year after year. The era of health and well-being, recognizing the importance of having and maintaining healthy staff with high energy levels, started in the 'Noughties'. Learning how to maximize and fully utilize the energy of staff is key to having organizations which can play a full role on the national and international stages.

Source: *Occupational Medicine*, Volume 68, Issue 4, June 2018, Page 254, https://doi.org/10.1093/occmed/kqx189. Copyright © The Author(s) 2018.

Fifty years ago: 'The shopworker'

Elizabeth Mitchell

The fascination of working in a shop lies in the fact that it is so closely connected with people. Their infinite needs can only be satisfied by many millions of individual meetings between customers and salesmen. In this career, every kind of person is involved. The salesman's success will depend upon his courtesy, and his ability to satisfy a 'want'. A customer must want something which he has bought—if an article is forced upon him by high-pressure salesmanship, he will subsequently regret the purchase, blame the shop and curse the salesman. The public have buying habits which vary, but in the main these are constant and can be predicted. But buying is also affected by local, national and international affairs. Fashions change, taxes are imposed overnight, and the retail trade must act as a shock-absorber until adjustments are made. Many criticize retail distribution as an unnecessary step in the progress of goods from the producer to the customer. The shopkeeper produces nothing—the goods leave the shop as they were received. He adds nothing but the price! Until the Industrial Revolution the shopkeeper was both producer and distributor—the farmer brought his produce to the market, the baker worked at the back of his house and sold his goods at the front. People lived on the products of their community. By 1850, thousands worked in factories producing goods in such abundance that they themselves could not have consumed them all even if they had had the opportunity to do so. Products, simple or complex, cheap or expensive, are worth nothing unless brought into contact with someone who desires them. As time passed, towns were joined by railways and products could be transported easily. The producer ceased to distribute and the distributor ceased to produce. This division of labour allowed the shop to make its contribution to our economic life. It is interesting to consider the work involved in running a shop. First there is the buying of the goods. These must be stored and an accurate record of stock kept. Advertising and display are necessary to promote the sale of the articles. These activities will necessitate payment of suppliers, giving of credit, cash control and despatching. Premises have to be kept clean and, last but not least, personnel cared for. These factors form the basic work pattern of retailing, and whether the shop is an enormous department store or a stall in the market, the same principles apply to both. In a big store, large numbers of people carry out these various functions. In Harrods, there is a working population of 5500, and only 1450 actually sell. A small shopkeeper must do everything himself. It showed singular lack of insight on the part of Napoleon when he sneeringly referred to us as a 'Nation of Shopkeepers'. We all know what the shopkeepers did to Napoleon.

Source: *Occupational Medicine*, Volume 68, Issue 4, June 2018, Page 261, https://doi.org/10.1093/occmed/kqx195. Copyright © The Author(s) 2018.

Originally from: The shopworker. *Trans Soc Occup Med* (1968) 18, 56–60.

Neurological memories

Anthony Seaton

One of my pleasures in reading journals is the stirring of memories, as when I read Dr Sealy's informative paper on the management of dizziness [1]. It started with a pithy quote from Dr WB Mathews' book, *Practical Neurology*, published in 1963. How well I remember it! At that time, as a young medical registrar, I was attracted to a career in neurology and obtained a post that gave me a great deal of practical experience of the subject. Indeed, there was rather more than I would have wished for, as my consultant's main interest was in his private practice and he expected me to do his clinics with the help of the house physician. I was familiar with the standard large textbooks of neurology but quickly found they were deficient in practical advice on management. Dr Mathews' book was a lifesaver, as it dealt with presenting symptoms rather than anatomical syndromes— headache, dizziness, blackouts, etc. I quickly became an adequate substitute for my boss.

Why did I not become a neurologist? It would certainly have become progressively easier as modern diagnostic techniques displaced carotid and vertebral angiograms, air encephalograms and frequent lumbar punctures, but it was not to be. I finally lost patience with my boss when he refused to come to his clinic to help me when my wife ran into difficulties in labour and I got my revenge by starting my outpatient letters with 'I saw your patient in the unexpected absence of Dr X'. It worked—he got a curt message from the professor of medicine, but I was instructed to change the format of my letters and when I refused he said: 'Don't ever ask me for a reference, Seaton!' So I went into cardiology then chest medicine and later added occupational medicine. In contrast, the house physician decided that medicine was not for him and became a knighted president of a surgical Royal College.

In my day one didn't train formally in medicine. It was necessary every year or so to apply for the jobs one thought appropriate, while in one's spare time (before study leave) one wrote papers, passed exams, tried to do research and taught medical students, activities which in that very competitive world increased one's chances of obtaining the jobs one wanted. My knowledge of cardiology led me to propose a hypothesis to explain the cardiac effects of air pollution and to delve into the effects of inhaled nanoparticles. My experience of chest medicine led me to propose an explanation for the increase in asthma in relation to maternal diet during pregnancy. My interest in neurology led me to studies of neurological effects of chemicals and to propose that significant exposures to solvents may have diverse effects on the nervous system depending on the genetic susceptibilities of the individual. And Dr Mathews' book inspired me to write with my colleagues a similar book for trainee occupational physicians, Practical Occupational Medicine. I hope you have a copy.

Reference

1. **Sealy A.** Vestibular assessment: a practical approach. *Occup Med (Lond)* 2014;**64**:78–86.

Source: *Occupational Medicine*, Volume 64, Issue 5, July 2014, Page 364, https://doi.org/10.1093/occmed/kqu059. Copyright © The Author 2014.

Consequences of OH alert syndrome

Karen Coomer

The three builders arrive and are soon working on various tasks like busy ants—I am the customer, it's my new house extension and the builder boss keeps me informed of every detail of the 'build' with a disproportionate amount of my time spent choosing bricks, tiles, windows and all that goes with a such a project. All good so far. The occupational health (OH) alert syndrome first kicks in when I notice the youngest builder wearing trainers and as my gaze wanders to three pairs of builder's feet—a variety of footwear is observed. I begin to see not just the building but the manual handling that goes with the construction, the ears not being protected when using noisy machinery, how the young one smokes and then puffs on his Ventolin inhaler, the preference for big sausage baps mid-morning instead of breakfast and the consumption of high-energy drinks throughout the day. I also listen as they compare blisters on their hands like a badge of honour, how their backs ache from lifting and handling and how the boss is clearly under pressure managing various projects. What to do? I resist the urge to inspect their hands for skin problems and carry out a spot spirometry test on the young one. I feel like a covert OH officer as I do daily dynamic risk assessments checking footwear, trying to sneak a look at their hands and put out fruit and suntan lotion with their tea—I realize it must look odd so I come clean and discuss with the boss my observations and what I do as a living. 'First time I've come across one of them', he replies. The next day I notice all three builders wearing safety boots, gloves and hearing protection and the young one is eating an apple. I feel an irrational sense of satisfaction but notice that they now look at me with a wary eye as I approach with the obligatory cups of tea. By the end of the project, the relationship moves from the role of important customer to counsellor as I listen in sound bites to the worries and woes of these builders whilst they drink their tea. It becomes increasingly difficult to get away; I'm becoming exhausted by this syndrome, can we ever be off duty as OH professionals? So, if anyone reading this appoints builders and the first thing they ask is whether you are one of those occupational health people you know that they have been exposed to a middle aged woman who takes an interest in safety footwear, likes to look at hands, puts apples on garden tables and eventually bribes her children to make builders tea.

Source: *Occupational Medicine*, Volume 65, Issue 4, June 2015, Page 289, https://doi.org/10.1093/occmed/kqu161. Copyright © The Author 2015.

Fifty years ago: 'Sickness absence resistance'

P.J. Taylor

Many doctors in industry make little or no attempt to study sickness absence, and the subject, despite its major economic importance, is one that is often considered as dull or unrewarding. This attitude is rationalized by the contention that the work involved is laborious and expensive, and sickness rates tend to be much the same from one year to the next. This short paper attempts to show that records which allow analysis of frequency distributions together with a study of men who appear to show a resistance to sickness absenteeism can be valuable in revealing the reasons for such behaviour. This in turn can provide indications how sickness absences may be controlled.

Details of sickness absence have been kept at this refinery for many years and since the sick pay scheme includes payment for short spells from one day upwards, all spells have been recorded. Although recent developments now allow all such records to be kept on magnetic tape and analysis to be done by a computer, there is still a lot to be said for a system which enables one to see at a glance the complete sickness record of any employee. The Seldex visible recording system is used and a card held for each employee.

In any one year, about 5% of the men are responsible for 25% of all spells of sickness absence in the refinery, while about 40% of the men have no spells at all. This type of distribution is not one of chance or at random, and it has been shown that for this refinery and other industrial groups, the distribution of sickness absence is consistently unequal and resembles that known to occur in injuries. The evidence thus suggests that for any one year, a phenomenon of sickness absence liability can be demonstrated. The sickness record cards also showed that the other extreme of behaviour can be measured, namely resistance to sickness absence. The proportion of hourly paid men having no such spell fell in an exponential manner with increasing years at risk but levelled off at about 4% after 12 years and showed a tendency to rise by 20 years.

To conclude in a somewhat light-hearted vein, an industrial medical officer is sometimes asked by a harassed personnel manager how absenteeism can be reduced. The results of this survey suggest that the following advice could be tendered. 'You should select men over 30 who claim to have had a wonderfully happy childhood, but may have marital problems. They should have a good attendance record in their previous employment and have no past history of peptic ulceration or nervous breakdown nor any lost time due to backache. They should not be troubled by constipation, but poor dental hygiene, bitten fingernails or a chronic physical condition are no bar to their employment. They should prefer to bicycle (or walk) to work where you should employ them on a continuous 3 cycle shift job where they will be happy and not long for promotion. Such men will not necessarily be better workers than others, but they will ease the pressure on the members of your department who record absenteeism, and on the sick pay fund.'

Source: *Occupational Medicine*, Volume 68, Issue 6, August 2018, Page 404, https://doi.org/10.1093/occmed/kqx197. Copyright © The Author(s) 2018.

Originally from: Sickness absence resistance. *Trans Soc Occup Med* (1968) 18, 96–100.

More hot air

Mike Gibson

At the RAF Institute of Aviation Medicine, we were used to receiving strange requests for advice and support. But the request from British Caledonian Airways (BCal) was unusual. They explained that when they established a new route, their pipe band went on the first scheduled flight to that destination and exited the aircraft playing. The trouble was that their new route was to Quito in Ecuador, at an altitude of 2850 m (9350 ft) above sea level; the executive who had negotiated the new route had collapsed whilst there and the company was concerned about the risk to members of their pipe band.

As I had recently reported some work to the Physiological Society on the respiratory stress of playing the bagpipes [1], I was directed to assist the Head of Breathing Systems Research Section, Dr AJF Macmillan, in investigating the issue. Theoretically, it should not have been a problem. But to make sure, BCal sent us two pipers to experiment on. Duly booted and spurred, they were installed in a decompression chamber (Figure 192.1) with me as safety medical officer and taken

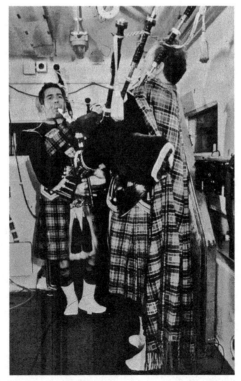

Figure 192.1 Pipers in the decompression chamber
Reproduced with permission from Gibson M. (2016). More hot air. *Occup Med (Lond)*. **66**(6):487. https://doi.org/10.1093/occmed/kqv210.

up to a simulated altitude of 9350 ft. The result was excruciating; the sound was akin to fingernails being dragged down a chalkboard. What none of us had taken into account was simple physics. The thinner air passed through the reeds more easily, altering the frequency of the notes by about a semitone. Our advice to the airline was two-fold: first, that the collapse was possibly the result of imbibing Canelazo—the traditional drink made using the local firewater (aguardiente); and second, that the band should pre-position to Quito and retune their pipes before meeting the first BCal flight to arrive. That is what happened, and no one collapsed.

Reference

1. **Harrison DK, Walker WF.** Micro-electrode measurement of skin pH in humans during ischaemia, hypoxia and local hypothermia. *J Physiol* 1979 Jun;**291**:339–50.

Source: *Occupational Medicine*, Volume 66, Issue 6, August 2016, Page 487, https://doi.org/10.1093/occmed/kqv210. Copyright © The Author 2016.

Internet addiction—caught in the web

Nerys Williams

The internet will soon have its 30th birthday. For years researchers have looked at internet addiction, specifically studying general compulsive use of the internet, cyber-stalking, excessive surfing and use of social media, playing games and internet gambling.

Back in 2002 Griffiths published a paper on the occupational health aspects of internet use [1] quoting their earlier work dating back to 1996 [2], proving that the issue is not new. Despite the intervening 22 years and vast growth of internet usage, we still don't read much about the topic in the UK health, safety and HR press.

This may be due to the lack of consensus on diagnosis and treatment of the condition or debate as to whether it actually exists. There is no formal definition or recognition of actual 'internet addiction' by established classification systems such as the Diagnostic and Statistical Manual (DSM) and the International Classification of Diseases (ICD). Internet gaming disorder was included for the first time in the appendix of DSM-V published in 2013 although there has been subsequent controversy. China, however, recognized internet addiction officially in 2008 and now reportedly runs 'boot camps' for the treatment of those affected [3].

Individuals who have problem usage have the same features of people suffering from other addictions: excessive or poorly controlled urges, preoccupations or behaviours which lead to distress. Practitioners report that they also experience symptoms salience, mood changes, tolerance and withdrawal.

There is also no consensus on a universally agreed standardized questionnaire to detect the condition; an estimated 21 instruments used for assessment are available [4], making like-for-like comparisons between studies impossible.

So it is not surprising that reported rates of internet 'addiction' are highly varied, with reported rates ranging from 0.8% in Italy [5] to 8.8% in Chinese adolescents [4]. Much higher rates are also reported, e.g. in another study of nearly 6500 Chinese 10–18-year olds, a rate of internet addiction of 26.5% was reported with a severe internet addiction rate of 0.96% [6].

Studies have shown that males are more frequently affected than females, younger people more than older and those with a high family income more than lower income groups. There are reported associations with impulsivity, neuroticism and loneliness, and a consistent association of co-morbid symptoms has also been reported. This is nothing new, a Taiwanese study, conducted over 10 years ago, found that female adolescents with internet addiction had higher attention deficit hyperactivity disorder symptoms and depressive disorders, while in males this was also seen but with additional higher rates of hostility [7]. Increased anxiety is also reported due to excessive social media use and the 'fear of missing out' (FOMO).

Occupational health professionals may be referred individuals undergoing disciplinary or performance procedures related to their prolonged/frequent internet use at work, hostility if they are denied computer access or debt due to gambling at work. Remembering that this could be a manifestation of a condition with all of the signs of addiction may assist in appropriate management.

References

1. **Griffiths MD.** Occupational health issues concerning Internet use in the workplace. *Work Stress* 2002;16.

2. **Griffiths MD.** Internet 'addiction': an issue for clinical psychology? *Clin Psychol Forum* **97**:32–36.

3. Inside the Chinese Boot Camp Treating Internet Addiction. http://telegraph.co.uk/news/health/11345412/Inside-the-Chinese-boot-camp-treating-internet-addicts (8 April 2018, date last accessed).

4. **Kuss DJ, Griffiths MD, Karila L, Billieux J.** Internet addiction: a systematic review of epidemiological research for the last decade. *Curr Pharm Des* 2014;**20**:4026–4052.

5. **Poli R, Agrimi E.** Internet addiction disorder: prevalence in an Italian student population. *Nord J Psychiatry* 2012;**66**:55–59.

6. **Xin M, Xing J, Pengfei W, Houru L, Mengcheng W, Hong Z.** Online activities, prevalence of Internet addiction and risk factors related to family and school among adolescents in China. *Addict Behav Rep* 2018;**7**:14–18.

7. **Yen JY, Ko CH, Yen CF, Wu HY, Yang MJ.** The comorbid psychiatric symptoms of Internet addiction: attention deficit and hyperactivity disorder (ADHD), depression, social phobia, and hostility. *J Adolesc Health* 2007;**41**:93–98.

Source: *Occupational Medicine*, Volume 68, Issue 7, October 2018, Page 468, https://doi.org/10.1093/occmed/kqy081. Copyright © The Author(s) 2018.

Hazard, risk and a bullet

John Challenor

Anything that might cause harm to a person is a hazard. Risk is the likelihood of that harm arising. One of the routinely hazardous activities that I undertake is motorcycling. Recently, I experienced a particularly hazardous assembly of events when I joined a group of like-minded enthusiasts on a charity fund-raising ride through Southern India (http://www.enduroindia.com/challenge.htm).

Unlike the ride, preparations were relatively leisurely—taking place over several months. During this period, there was time to undertake several long-distance mixed terrain practice rides, which included on and off road motorcycling on and around Salisbury Plain (http://www. trailandoffroad.co.uk/Home.html). There was also time to evaluate various types and styles of personal protective equipment (PPE), update my vaccination status and test drive anti-malarial tablets.

I viewed and reviewed films of previous enduro rides on the Enduro India website and took careful note of the climate, terrain and PPE worn by participants. Excellent support and comprehensive checklists were provided by the organizers who were enthusiastic and encouraging. Even the type and style of bike we would all be riding was familiar to me as I owned a Royal Enfield Bullet. But my fertile imagination had not prepared me for the sensual and physical challenges of the event itself. The heat and smell of over 60 revving motorbike engines on the first day would be an unforgettable memory.

The experience of riders ranged from absolute beginners who had taken their motorbike tests specifically for the event to superbike riders, who regularly attended track days. Ages ranged from those in their third decade to their ninth decade of life; those of us past retirement age surely demonstrating the survivor effect. Daily safety and planning meetings were detailed and thorough. Nevertheless risks were ever present and every minute of every hour of every day presented a skidpan full of thrills, spills, falls, collisions, and examples of momentary lapses of concentration. For some riders, these were trivial, embarrassing, and merely inconvenient; for others, injurious and extremely painful. For one rider, his significant event was sadly fatal. I witnessed them all.

The organizers were quick to identify dangerous practices and lost little time in naming and shaming perpetrators. From a field of over 60 bikes travelling over 1400 miles, about 15% were involved in 'incidents'. The most serious were near misses and collisions with vehicles and animals. All riders were aware of the ever-present chaotic and undisciplined driving/riding behaviour around us and that we should expect the unexpected. A few of us wondered at the time whether some of the group were riding beyond their ability and were courting disaster. Was the hazard and risk perception of those involved in mishaps different to those who completed the ride without incident?

Did I think it was worth it? Yes, but I feel concern for those who were injured and I grieve for Chris, who swerved to avoid a cow and collided with oncoming traffic. Was he killed by his own Bullet?

Source: *Occupational Medicine*, Volume 61, Issue 7, October 2011, Page 479, https://doi.org/10.1093/occmed/kqr091. Copyright © The Author 2011.

Anti-smoking legislation

Mike Gibson

Tobacco was introduced to Europe in 1493 when Columbus returned from his first voyage to the New World. Tobacco leaves and instruction in their use had been given to some of his crew by Tainos Indians on Hispaniola. Smoking and the use of tobacco gradually took hold although it was initially the preserve of the rich. Pipe-smoking was introduced to the UK in 1572 by Sir Francis Drake. By 1590, tobacco use was such a problem in mainland Europe that Pope Urban VII threatened to excommunicate anyone who 'took tobacco in the porchway of, or inside, a church, whether by chewing it, smoking it with a pipe, or sniffing it in powdered form through the nose'. Ten years later, Samuel Rowlands wrote in Epigram 18 of 'The Letting of Humours in the Head-Vaine':

'... Death only stabs the heart and so life ends: But this same poyson, steeped India weed, In head, hart, lungs, doth soote & cobwebs breed. With that he gasp'd, & breath'd out such a smoke, That all the standers by were like to choke.'

In 1604, King James VI and I issued his 'Counterblaste to Tobacco' which contains the oft-quoted passage '... a custom loathsome to the eye, hateful to the nose, harmful to the brain, dangerous to the lungs, and in the black stinking fume thereof nearest resembling the horrible Stygian smoke of the pit that is bottomless.'

From then on, successive governments have been caught between two conflicting demands: to restrict smoking and to maximize income from taxing tobacco. Excise duty on tobacco was first introduced in 1660 and currently raises over £12bn a year. On the other hand, restrictions include the banning of smoking in the chamber of the House of Commons in 1693 and the introduction of smoke-free carriages on British railways in 1868. Following the work of Doll and Hill [1] and the 1962 Royal College of Physicians report on smoking and health, there has been a stream of legislation restricting tobacco advertising and availability, of which The Tobacco and Related Products Regulations 2016 (SI 2016/507) is the latest. One of the most important laws is The Health Act 2006 (c28) (and similar legislation in Northern Ireland, Scotland and Wales) which prohibited smoking in the workplace.

There have been various sanctions imposed for breach of these laws. A man has been fined £200 for not displaying a No Smoking sign in a brand new company van he was collecting. At least one person has been fined for smoking in a car with children present. Another man has been jailed recently for discarding a cigarette in an aeroplane toilet, causing a fire.

But who was the first person to be imprisoned for smoking? Rodrigo de Jerez, a member of Columbus' crew, was imprisoned in 1493 for 7 years by the Inquisition who determined that only the Devil could have taught him to blow smoke out of his mouth and nose.

Reference

1. **Doll R, Hill AB.** Smoking and carcinoma of the lung. *Br Med J* 1950;2:739–748.

Source: *Occupational Medicine*, Volume 67, Issue 8, November 2017, Page 640, https://doi.org/10.1093/occmed/kqx104. Copyright © The Author 2017.

Fifty years ago: 'Productivity, morale and occupational medicine'

John Garnett

The Industrial Society, both recently and previously when it was the Industrial Welfare Society, has had close contacts with occupational medical officers and has done what it can to encourage industry and commerce to pay attention to this aspect of their business. It is a highly practical society, now specializing in promoting the best use of human resources. Before becoming Director of the Industrial Society, the speaker had been for 15 years on the sales side and on the personnel side of a large chemical company, and it was from his observations during this 20-year period that he was talking. He had often wondered why more companies did not appoint full-time medical officers and pay more attention to what these people could achieve for industry. There are still many large companies running on industrial nurses only. Was this, at least in part, because medical officers were paying attention to human problems in far too narrow a way? What is the problem? The main problem in industry today is not the over-exploitation of people, but their under-use; failure to motivate them, to get them to accept that their work matters and that they are needed. One finds this among the young as well as among the more senior, where the job may have outgrown them and they are left utterly frustrated. This is reflected in blood pressures, thromboses, sickness absence and lateness. All this is not helped by the need for large units and the fact that much work, whether we like it or not, will continue to be boring, many of the modern jobs being worse than the old. The answers do not lie in money, which may increase the problem rather than decrease it, nor with the unions, who do not carry the responsibility for motivating people, nor with welfare above a certain level. As the State improves the basic welfare of the nation with better medical services, sickness schemes, pension funds and recreation clubs, medical centres in industry are less necessary than they were. Where do the answers lie and what can Occupational Medical Officers do to help?

Some of the key strengths of the industrial medical officer are that he is a man of professional integrity with a greater loyalty to the profession than to himself or his company. He is also a highly technical person associated with life and death. He is known to be deeply concerned with the individual. In all these respects, he has a particular ability to influence management, if only he will bring his influence to bear on the all-important matters of man management as well as on physical environment. Of course, whatever time is available is not enough, but might not some greater part of it be best allocated to walking the job and bringing home to management and supervision that the way to lead men and organize their leadership can have a more profound effect on health and well-being than any glamorous equipment in a medical department?

Source: *Occupational Medicine*, Volume 68, Issue 8, November 2018, Page 511, https://doi.org/10.1093/occmed/kqx199. Copyright © The Author(s) 2018.

Originally from: Productivity, morale and occupational medicine. *Trans Soc Occup Med* (1968) **18**, 120–121. Available at: *Occup Med (Lond)* 1968;**18**:120–121. DOI: 10.1093/occmed/18.2.120

Corbett McDonald

John Hobson

Corbett McDonald, one of the truly colossal figures in occupational health, died in 2016. In 'Farewell to Corbett, but Not to His Contributions' Trevor Ogden and Graham Gibbs commemorate the first anniversary of his death in the Annals of Workplace Exposures and Health [1].

John Corbett McDonald was born in Belfast in April 1918. He qualified at St Mary's Hospital Medical School, was an army medical officer during World War II and then trained in public health at the London School of Hygiene and Tropical Medicine and at Harvard University. He became director of the Epidemiological Research Laboratory at the Public Health Laboratory at Colindale in 1960 before moving to chair the new Department of Epidemiology and Health at McGill University in Montreal in 1964. Together with Dr Christopher Wagner, newly arrived from the Pneumoconiosis Research Unit near Cardiff, he began his research interest in asbestos. Funding was obtained from the asbestos industry at a time when such funding for research was not unusual. In a retrospective cohort study of 11 000 Quebec chrysotile miners and millers born between 1891 and 1920, they found excess lung cancer deaths at 'extremely high dust exposure', but little or no excess below levels 'orders of magnitude higher than permitted today'. In 1972, Corbett advised the International Agency for Research on Cancer which concluded that all commercial types of asbestos could cause lung cancer. Whilst his work was one of the major studies that contributed to understanding the risk of asbestos disease, Corbett was publicly attacked by those who disagreed with his findings and the use made of them by the asbestos industry. This assault lasted for most of Corbett's lifetime and threatened to overshadow his other considerable contributions to occupational health. He initiated a series of occupational disease surveillance schemes including respiratory diseases (SWORD) and skin diseases amongst others. He worked on sick building syndrome, solvent exposure and psychiatric disorders, chemical exposure and congenital defects and spontaneous abortion. He studied flour and other aeroallergens, silica in potteries and cryptogenic fibrosing alveolitis. During his career he was head of the TUC Centenary Institute of Occupational Health at the London School of Hygiene and Tropical Medicine and Professor Emeritus of Clinical Epidemiology at the National Heart and Lung Institute.

Corbett remained active well into old age despite losing a leg after being hit by a motorcycle. He authored over 70 of his 319 papers after his 70th birthday, the last one appearing in the Annals in 2010 when he was 92. At the age of 93 he made several visits to Bangladesh where he helped set up a postgraduate training scheme and worked on the effects of arsenic contamination of drinking water. However, even in his eighties, Corbett's personal integrity was attacked and demands made for McGill University to investigate his research. Finally and eventually the Research Integrity Officer of McGill concluded that 'there is no evidence that the design of the research, its conduct, and its reporting was influenced by the industry'.

Reference

1. **Ogden T, Gibbs G**. Farewell to Corbett, but not to his contributions. *Ann Work Expo Health* 2017;**61**:499–503. doi:10.1093/annweh/wxx013.

Shale is here again

Anthony Seaton

The current enthusiasm for fracking takes me back to the oil crisis of the late 1970s. I had been asked to see a post-thoracotomy patient and, when he recovered, found that his lesion had been pneumoconiotic. When I enquired which mine he worked in, he told me that it had been a shale mine and since Hunter's old textbook stated that pneumoconiosis didn't occur in shale miners, I did a little trawl round the local hospital's pathology department, found some other cases, wrote them up and, knowing that the USA was opening up its massive shale oil reserves and interested in possible adverse health effects, applied for a grant to the US Department of Energy to study the risks of shale oil production. One patient turned into a research programme!

Occupational physicians will recall the story of the oil shale industry to the west of Edinburgh established in the 1850s by James Young, the production of the first mineral oil and the discovery of the second known cause of cancer, among the paraffin workers in West Lothian and later among the cotton spinners of Lancashire. The grant allowed us to study the workers in the Scottish oil shale industry in 1983–84, 30 years after the industry had closed, including their mortality and, among survivors, the risks of skin and lung disease. The results were used to provide risk estimates for the developing US shale industry.

In the course of this study, I was able to visit the developing mines in Colorado and was interested to see what must have been the first attempts to obtain the oil without having to send miners down to bring up the shale, using explosives and *in situ* methods for extraction. Of course, we were familiar with the production of gas from coal in the UK prior to the opening of the North Sea industry and British Coal was at that time experimenting with *in situ* production of oil from the coal deposits. Alas this advanced work was curtailed as the UK coal industry was decimated through the 1980s.

Recently, I was telling a retired Yorkshire coal miner something of the Scottish oil shale industry and he remarked that in his pit, there had been so much gas that it was put to use to heat the mine buildings. And, of course, we all know that methane is an ever-present hazard in mining. The Scottish shale industry, which made oil from stone, hence *petroleum*, was eventually put out of business by the discovery of liquid oil deposits in the USA, discovered while drilling for gas, hence *gasoline*. Now the writing is on the wall for the coal industry and soon may be for the oil industry with fracking and eventually, thanks to an increasing awareness of the changing climate, even for the gas industry. But those two synonyms, petrol and gas, will remind our grandchildren of the greedy exploitation of the world's fossil fuels that led to the uncomfortable world that they will live in.

Source: *Occupational Medicine*, Volume 64, Issue 8, December 2014, Page 588, https://doi.org/10.1093/occmed/kqu116. Copyright © The Author 2014.

Index